This book is due for return on or before the last date shown below.

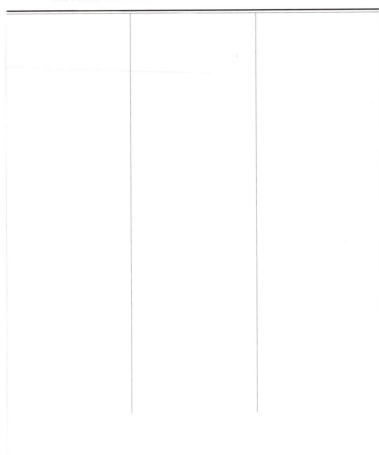

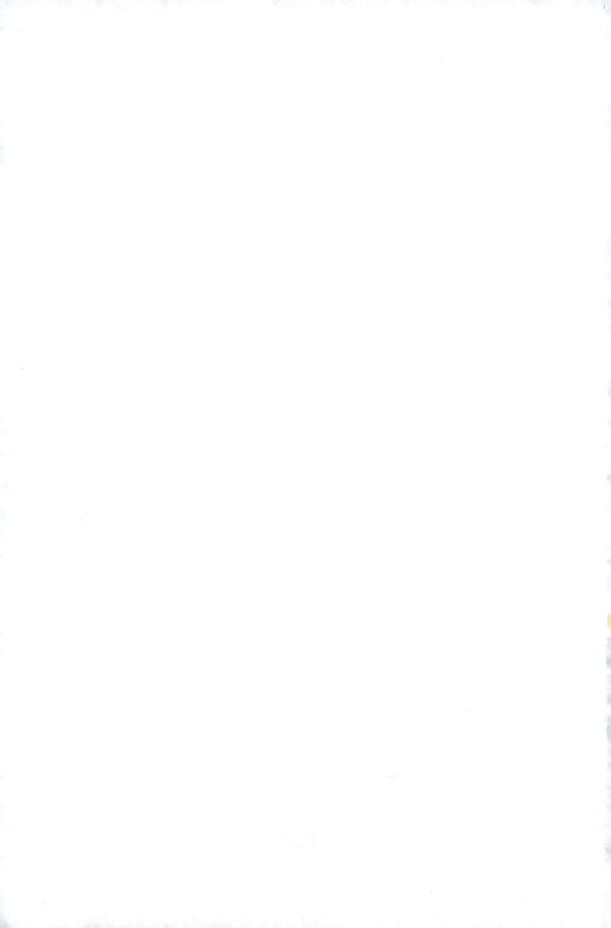

MBA for Medics

EMMA STANTON

and

CLAIRE LEMER

Foreword by
PROFESSOR SIR LIAM DONALDSON
*Chief Medical Officer for England
(1998–2010)*

Radcliffe Publishing
Oxford • New York

Radcliffe Publishing Ltd
18 Marcham Road
Abingdon
Oxon OX14 1AA
United Kingdom

www.radcliffepublishing.com
Electronic catalogue and worldwide online ordering facility.

British Library Cataloguing in Publication Data

A catalogue record for this book is available from the British Library.

ISBN-13: 978 184619 438 2

Typeset by Pindar NZ, Auckland, New Zealand
Printed and bound by Cadmus Communications, USA

Contents

Foreword

Travelling abroad, the British are not famed for their linguistic ability. There is a stereotype of a slightly hapless English man trying, red-faced, to make a simple purchase in a shop somewhere on the European continent. Through the medium of wild gesticulation and slow, frustrated, repetitive shouting, he may or may not make himself understood and get what he wants. The view is a stereotypical one. It is grossly unfair to the many who speak foreign languages well. But often it is true.

When two people meet and cannot converse, the result is often misunderstanding – not just of the conversation's content, but also of one another. Each leaves with a lesser opinion of the other. Mistrust and stereotype are bred. The next time either encounters another of the same tribe, his ability to conduct a useful interaction is impaired.

Those who immerse themselves in learning a foreign language have a far more pleasurable experience. They learn a new vocabulary. More, they come to know a new people, a new culture, a new view of the world. When they converse with native speakers, the experience is often positive on both sides. Both parties can leave a conversation having learnt something from the other. Trust begins to be sewn.

Every profession has its own language and culture. The medical profession is by no means an exception. Not just in a shared jargon, in Greek, Latin and acronyms, but also in approach, mindset, and culture. Doctors have a particular way of thinking and communicating. The language of healthcare management is different. It shares the same alphabet and the same syntax, but many of the words are different. When words are shared with the language of clinical medicine, their meaning may not be. Healthcare managers can happily converse amongst themselves. Doctors can converse amongst themselves. The problem can come when the two groups meet.

Increasingly, doctors are seeing the value of learning the language of management. Not just its words, but its view on the world, its approach, its great strengths. A number of doctors have learnt the language and skills by gaining a formal qualification such as an MBA. Many more have followed an experiential route.

This book is for doctors who see the value that an education in management can bring, whether formal or informal. It is for those who seek to speak both languages. It is especially for those who wish to become part of both tribes – perhaps hoping that any tribal divide that they may currently observe will one day cease to exist.

In a sense, the book reflects the authors' own journeys from the world of medicine to the world of management, to a world that combines the two. Becoming bilingual is enjoyable, empowering and highly valuable. The prize is not conversation in foreign lands, but fluent engagement with people who work in the same building. Doctors may enjoy the journey, but it is patients for whom this book really matters. When doctors are engaged with the management and leadership of clinical services, the bar is raised towards higher quality, safer care. The ultimate reason for doctors to be ambitious and to gain a management education is not for personal gain or for more letters after their name, but for the prize of better, safer healthcare for patients.

Sir Liam Donaldson
Chief Medical Officer for England (1998–2010)
July 2010

Preface

Well, here's another *nice* mess you've got me into.

Oliver Hardy to Stan Laurel

This book is the result of remarkable tenacity and endurance, matched only by over-enthused optimism. The book developed from a series of conversations between the authors. It is a testament to the 'power of we' over I. Without the partnership between the authors this book would not have been possible – the fear of the blank page, not to mention NHS accounts, would have been overwhelming. When we look to healthcare, we observe that successful leadership is not infrequently the result of similar partnerships. It is as an encouragement to others of the values of developing such teamwork that we begin this book.

Many books already exist about MBAs. So why did we feel the need to write another one?

Well, during the course of our studies, many clinicians have approached us with intrepid curiosity to discuss whether an MBA is for them. However, the time and financial barriers for MBAs are substantial and insurmountable for most. As a qualification, let us state from the outset that an MBA is not a requirement for success in either the healthcare or the corporate world. Although the title of the book suggests it is targeted solely at the medical profession, it has been written for all those interested in learning more about the use of an MBA for the world of healthcare, not just doctors.

Furthermore, this book is not a self-contained Masters in Business Administration. It does not include everything that is on an MBA syllabus but we have included references for further reading at the end of every chapter. This book's aim is threefold: to encourage medics to think about management and business; to provide key insights for those whose interest is already piqued; and lastly, preparation for those wanting to go forth and study for an MBA to assist them to do so.

Throughout the book we have tried to bring alive the issues discussed by using an imaginary hospital St Anywhere. This medium sized District General Hospital is meant to epitomise standard hospital care in the NHS, and allows clinicians to relate what they are learning back to patient care.

The current turbulent context to reduce spend on healthcare requires strategic leadership and decision-making. This text provides a succinct summary targeted at clinicians in or preparing for leadership roles. We are confident that the value of an MBA is in the tools it brings to a clinicians' skill set. Such a blend of skills confronts the economic challenge head on, enabling clinicians to work alongside managers, to increase both quality and productivity, to ultimately bring 'value' to healthcare.

Emma Stanton
Claire Lemer
July 2010

About the authors

Dr Emma Stanton is a Psychiatry Specialist Registrar. From 2008–10, Emma was seconded as a Clinical Advisor to the Chief Medical Officer at the Department of Health, including a secondment to Bupa Health Dialog. From 2010–11, Emma is a Harkness Fellow in Health Policy in the USA, researching how to measure and improve the value of mental healthcare. Emma co-edited *Clinical Leadership: Bridging the divide* (Quay Books, 2009). She became interested in leadership and teamwork after competing in the Round the World Yacht Race 2005–06. Emma is passionate about clinicians developing management and leadership skills from an early stage in their training. In 2006, Emma was a founding member and has subsequently Chaired BAMMbino, the junior doctors' arm of the British Association of Medical Managers. In 2009, Emma was appointed as an Emerging Leader to the National Leadership Council, chaired by the Chief Executive of the NHS. Emma has an MBA from Imperial College, London. Her dissertation included learning about patient safety from analogous high hazard industries. Emma is a Founder and Director of Diagnosis, clinical leadership social enterprise.

Dr Claire Lemer works both as a Paediatric Registrar in North London and as Operations Manager for Ophthalmology, in an adjacent hospital. Claire co-edited *Clinical Leadership: Bridging the divide* (Quay Books, 2009). She developed an interest in management as a result of spending two and a half years at the Department of Health and WHO working for the Chief Medical Officer. During this time Claire developed her interest in quality improvement and patient safety and helped set up a leadership scheme for young doctors, 'The CMO's Clinical Advisor Scheme'. In 2004–05 Claire was a Commonwealth Fund/Health Foundation Harkness Fellow in Health Policy, based in Boston at Brigham and Women's Hospital, where she researched the effects of communication in paediatric medication safety. Claire has an MD, from University of London, an MPH from Harvard and has recently completed an MBA from Oxford. Claire is a Founder and Director of Diagnosis.

Boxes, tables and figures

BOXES

TABLES

FIGURES

Acknowledgements

Two roads diverged in a wood – I took the road less travelled, and that
has made all the difference.

Robert Frost, 'The Road Not Taken' (1916)

Throughout our careers, from time to time we have taken the road less travelled.
Doing so has been made possible by the support and mentoring of other senior
medical managers including Professor Sir Liam Donaldson, Sir Cyril Chantler and
Professor Jenny Simpson. Throughout their careers, these trailblazers have pioneered
the importance of equipping doctors with management and leadership skills alongside their clinical training, to provide the best possible care for patients. In addition,
they have nurtured and welcomed those more junior to them, and that has made
all the difference.

We completed our MBAs at Imperial College Business School, London, and Saïd
Business School, Oxford, in 2009. We are grateful for the lecturers and peers who
taught us. These degrees laid the foundations for this book. This book is enhanced
by the personal stories of many doctors who have also completed MBAs. We thank
them for sharing their experiences.

Emma and Claire met on the Prepare to Lead mentorship scheme organised and
inspired by Oliver Warren under the auspices of NHS London. The scheme gave us
both incredible opportunities that we might otherwise never have managed, but
most importantly it brought together kindred slightly maverick spirits who gained
from finding each other. So our thanks go to both Oliver Warren and NHS London
for supporting the innovative scheme.

Finally, we would like to thank Dr James Mountford for his counsel, and our
families for their brilliant support.

Emma and Claire

Authors' note

Healthcare practice and knowledge is constantly changing and developing as new research and treatments, changes in procedures, drugs and equipment become available. The authors and publisher have, as far as possible, taken care to confirm that the information contained complies with the latest standards of practice and legislation.

Never doubt that a small group of thoughtful,
committed citizens can change the world.
Indeed, it is the only thing that ever has.

MARGARET MEAD

SECTION 1

From good to great

In his 2001 classic book *Good to Great*, Jim Collins seeks to answer the question, 'Can a good company become a great company and, if so, how?'

Together with his team, he examined 1435 Fortune 500 companies. Of these, only 11 met all of the criteria for transforming from good to great, demonstrating just how difficult making this leap is. In the book, the discipline of 'first who' emphasises the importance of having the 'right people' in key positions. The text presses the importance of character attributes over specialised skills, which can be learnt.

An MBA is one way of learning skills and acquiring knowledge. However, achieving an MBA alone does not guarantee you will progress from being a good to great leader. This first section of the book considers the evidence for doing an MBA and discusses the alternative options.

FURTHER READING

Collins J (2001). *Good to Great*. London: Random House Business Books.

CHAPTER 1

So, why do an MBA?

Leadership and learning are indispensible to each other.

John F Kennedy (1917–63)

INTRODUCTION

A Masters in Business Administration (MBA) is the world's most popular postgraduate degree programme. Every year, in the United States of America, over 90 000 students graduate with MBAs. In the United Kingdom, over 10 000 MBA students graduate annually. Yet in the UK, only a handful of these are also medically qualified.

When fellow clinicians learn that we have an MBA, the ensuing question is not infrequently: 'So, what was your Masters in?' Amongst the reams of qualifications collected by doctors, an MBA has not yet become mainstream currency; maybe it never will.

This book doesn't set out to advocate or endorse MBAs for medics. It aims to present an overview for the individual to decide if it is the right career path for them. This opening chapter sets the scene by exploring the current relevance of the MBA and the applicability of it for healthcare professionals.

WHAT IS AN MBA?

The first MBA programme was developed in America in the early 1900s. It was introduced to Europe in the 1960s. Nowadays, with thousands of universities offering MBA programmes around the world, there are increasingly flexible ways of learning, as discussed in Chapter 4.

In summary, an MBA covers all of the functions and practices of a business, i.e. commercial activity. Historically, MBAs have focused on delivering the core subjects of accounting, finance, human resources and marketing. These subjects form the foundation of most MBA programmes. An overview of these areas is provided in Section 2 of this book. MBAs have subsequently evolved to include 'softer' areas such as leadership, entrepreneurialism, sustainability, risk, globalisation and ethics. These subjects are often included as 'elective' modules on MBAs, offering scope and flexibility to cater for individual preferences. Studying for an MBA inevitably serves to broaden horizons, open doors and create new opportunities.

MBAs AND THE CORPORATE WORLD

In an analysis and ranking of the performance of 2000 CEOs (Chief Executive Officers) globally, CEOs with an MBA ranked 40 places higher on average than CEOs who didn't have an MBA. Whilst this connection demonstrates association, it doesn't infer causation between doing an MBA and becoming a CEO.

Over the last year, the reputation of MBAs has been attacked for their role on the ethical and strategic lapses that led to the 'credit crunch'. In response to the criticisms that MBA programmes focus too extensively on creating shareholder value through high-risk strategies with insufficient emphasis on sustainable practices and stakeholder responsibility, the Association of MBAs carried out an extensive review of MBAs (Durham, 2009). This survey – of over 100 business schools – identified that the top three reasons for individuals doing MBAs were:

➤ career progression (39%)
➤ career change (28%)
➤ gain more detailed knowledge/improve skills (18%).

These reasons are likely to resonate with medics considering studying an MBA. Section 4 of this book explores career opportunities both in and out of the NHS for medics with MBAs.

In addition, the survey showed that nearly one-quarter of MBA graduates were self-employed (23%). The two largest business sectors represented amongst MBA graduates were consulting (15%) and finance (13%). Healthcare, together with the pharmaceutical industry, accounted for only 6% of MBA alumni. Consulting and finance may be overrepresented on MBA programmes, as certain career paths in these sectors require an MBA for progression. However, for most sectors, including healthcare, doing an MBA comes down to proactive individuals writing business cases to convince their line managers to invest in their development to do an MBA.

Across Europe, women make up 30% of MBA students yet remain largely absent from the top positions of large corporations, as in healthcare organisations. Only 10% of board members of FTSE 100 companies are women (*The Times*, 2010). By means of introduction, FTSE is an independent company jointly owned by the *Financial Times* and the London Stock Exchange. It provides objective information and ranking about commercial markets.

The options for MBA programmes study are increasingly global. The 2010 UK business school performance rankings for MBAs are listed in the following chapter. Reflecting increasingly globalised economies, MBAs frequently include international case studies and study tours. From personal experience, the international MBA study tour was a highlight of the MBA, both socially and for learning purposes.

On the social theme, one of the most advantageous and implicitly intangible benefits not explicitly stated in any MBA curricula is the personal networks derived from participating in such programmes. The concept of networks and networking is discussed further in Chapter 7. Many doctors may feel uncomfortable with the concept of 'networking with a purpose' but this is largely due to unfamiliarity with it as a skill. The importance of networking cannot be undervalued. *Connected* (2010), by Christakis and Fowler, describes how social networks shape our lives and influence what we do. If you are considering changing or upgrading your role or career then the advantage of an MBA is that it exposes you to a broad range of completely unrelated industries and opportunities. Similarly for those already committed to a new career trajectory, doing an MBA helps to identify kindred spirits.

To maximise your MBA experience, many business schools provide accompanying Executive Coaching alongside the degree. This personal developmental opportunity is rarely available in the public sector. It can make an enormous difference to crystallising thought processes about career development and next steps.

Not all are advocates of MBA programmes. Amongst others, Mintzberg is a well-known critic of MBAs and challenges the evidence that such courses proffer benefit to students. Mintzberg notably argues that MBA courses focus too much on the academic aspects or the 'science of management' and fail to focus on the art of management. Mintzberg believes that management is a craft that cannot easily be taught, but rather has to be learned from experience or at least analysis of experiences. Mintzberg gives his support to courses that take those with real world experience and help them to build and reflect on this, rather than MBA programmes. His concern surrounds the clear trend that MBA programmes are increasingly geared towards those just graduating from first degrees with limited or no real-world experience and who all too often do an MBA for the 'stamp on the CV' value.

MBAs AND MEDICINE

In the UK, 17% of public spending in 2009 was spent on healthcare. This is more than that spent on education (13%). The proportional share of UK gross domestic product (GDP) spent on healthcare is set to rise to 14% by 2030. Both the level of spending and the rate of increase in healthcare spend in the UK are unsustainable for the future economy. At present, the National Health Service (NHS) is battling with the two-fold challenge of improving the quality of healthcare whilst simultaneously improving overall productivity. As long as the quality of care is perceived as the sole responsibility of the clinician, and productivity is perceived as resting entirely within the managers' domain, both aims are compromised.

One of the solutions proposed to close the yawning divide between clinicians and healthcare managers is to implement interdisciplinary education from an early stage in training. This would enable a greater mutual understanding of professional cultures. Joint initiatives, such as combining managerial and clinical reporting, aim to identify system failures at an earlier stage to prevent recurrences of the tragic sequence of events at the Bristol Royal Infirmary (1995) and more recently at Mid Staffordshire NHS Trust (2009).

In the US, nearly one-third of medical colleges offer a formal integrated degree in medicine (MD) in combination with a business school. The five-year Harvard MD/MBA programme was created in 2005 specifically to develop clinical leaders. Students concentrate on medicine for the first two years with a management internship in a hospital or healthcare organisation in between. In the third year, students continue medical training as well as doing several management courses, including looking directly at management problems on the wards. During the fourth year, students do an MBA with a clinical rotation and in their fifth year students complete their MBA and clinical rotations. Such programmes aim to produce doctors bilingual in both medical and 'management speak' who can act as cross-cultural agents narrowing the gap between doctors and managers. The majority of graduates from this programme enter clinical roles. It is too soon to measure the success and ability of these graduates in rising to healthcare leadership positions.

There are many more medically qualified chief executives in the US than in the UK. This is a likely consequence of fundamental differences in healthcare funding and ensuing fragmented infrastructure. This has pushed clinicians in America into developing commercial acumen. At present, no undergraduate medical curricula include MBAs in the UK. However, some medical schools offer intercalated Masters in Healthcare Management, discussed in Chapter 2.

In the UK, MBAs have historically been designed to attract students with five to ten years' postgraduate experience. For doctors, this typically means doing MBA post-membership exams. This timing aims to enrich classroom discussion based on real-life experience. Across Europe, the average age of a student on a full-time MBA programme is 27 years. For those studying part-time or via distance learning, it is 34 years. Undertaking an MBA at a later stage in your career can be a more strategic move to achieve a promotion or career change.

Financial cost is a significant barrier to many medics pondering on whether to do an MBA. However, there are sources of funding available, as discussed in Chapter 6. In addition to cost, MBAs are a huge time commitment. Even executive or part-time MBAs can demand an additional 10–20 hours study a week, as well as lecture attendance. For medics, this is on top of years of ploughing through medical exams as well as hoovering up other research qualifications, all while balancing the commitments of an on-call rota. At the end of it, there are no guarantees that doing an MBA will lead to a promotion or even recognition in healthcare. In fact, there is a risk that it may even be perceived pejoratively as 'going over to the dark side'. Currently, the low numbers of NHS clinical consultants with MBAs, mean that there are few role models to encourage trainees to consider this as a desirable option.

The majority of NHS consultants are 'baby boomers' (aged up to 62). Findings from research into the attitudes and behaviour of 'Generation Y' (individuals under 30) suggest that if 'Gen Y' are not being given what they need at work, they will leave. The concept of a 'job for life' is no longer relevant for medicine or elsewhere. This means that doctors are likely to be increasingly looking to develop transferable commercially applicable skills. As such, an MBA may offer additional skills to compliment clinical training, for employment avenues outlined in the final chapter.

SUMMARY

With global healthcare demand predicted to rise, there is a need for healthcare to learn from the corporate sector about how best to improve quality alongside improvements in productivity. Medics doing MBAs is one possible route for cross-sector innovation and learning to achieve this.

In addition to the wider healthcare policy considerations, the individual commitment and ultimate value of an MBA rests with how much you are prepared to invest of yourself and the quality of teaching you receive. This makes where and how you do your MBA key considerations in the value derived, discussed in Chapter 3.

If success is about the combination of knowledge and experience, then an MBA will not guarantee making you a great leader but may very well enhance a potential one. Although not relevant for all, an MBA can be considered a significant landmark on an aspiring individual's leadership journey.

The range of possible career options outlined in the concluding section of this book may be useful incentives to consider when deciding on an MBA. However, it is important to appreciate that many of these are achievable without an MBA. Alternative academic options to an MBA are considered in the following chapter.

FURTHER READING

Association of MBAs. Available at: www.mbaworld.com

Christakis NA, Fowler J (2010). *Connected: amazing power of social networks and how they shape our lives*. New York: HarperPress.

Durham Business School and Association of MBAs (2009). *The Post Downturn MBA: An Agenda for Change*. London: Association of MBAs.

Hansen M, Ibarra H (20 January 2010). Does an MBA make you a better CEO? *Harvard Business Review* (The Conversation blog). Available at: http://blogs.hbr.org/cs/2010/01/does_an_mba_make_you_a_better.html (accessed 18 June 2010).

James J, Bibb S, Walker S (2008). *Generation Y: what they want from work*. A summary report of the 'Tell it how it is' research. London: Talentsmoothie. Available at: www.talentsmoothie.com/wp-content/uploads/2009/12/TIHIS-report-Summary-and-Conclusion.pdf (accessed 18 June 2010).

Nash D (2003). Doctors and managers: mind the gap. *BMJ*; **326**: 652–3.

Senior A (11 March 2010). Why women are such bad networkers. *The Times*. Available at: http://women.timesonline.co.uk/tol/life_and_style/women/article7057300.ece (accessed 18 June 2010).

Stephenson J (2009). Getting down to business. *BMJ*; **339**: b4595.

CHAPTER 2

Alternatives to an MBA

It does not matter whether the cat is black or white. What matters is that it catches mice.

Deng Xiaoping (1904–97)

INTRODUCTION

Flowing on from the foundation laid in the previous chapter, this chapter discusses the alternative options for formal management training, beyond doing an MBA. There is a growing choice available for healthcare professionals interested in gaining management experience or skills.

Due to the constantly changing landscape, this chapter is not exhaustive. It aims to ensure that those considering an MBA have at least a working knowledge of alternative options, which can be looked at in more detail if desired.

BACKGROUND

Many argue that, as with the other industries, the best training for management is experience. A recent study of 22 medical chief executives in the NHS identifies that the old chestnut 'see one, do one, teach one' applies as much to clinicians entering management roles as it does to clinical practice. The majority of these medical chief executives learnt their skills 'on the job'. With the increasing complexity and demands of healthcare delivery, the consensus is that leadership roles are no longer appropriate or accessible for 'enthusiastic amateurs'. MBAs, amongst other courses, contain skills and information that can facilitate good management practice, and provide the confidence to step into roles where experience can be garnered, thus presenting the case for taught programmes to be part of aspiring leaders' preparation.

To date, a mixed response seems to be unfolding. Strategic Health Authorities under the auspices and in part funded by the Department of Health and encouraged by the National Leadership Council, are developing a set of innovative programmes for providing clinicians with such skills. Much investment has gone into junior doctors' leadership development through programmes such as the Darzi Fellowship Scheme in the London Deanery. Such schemes give trainees the opportunity to learn in an experiential style about quality improvement and healthcare management. Of note though is that many, if not the majority, prefer to combine their practical hands-on learning with a more structured programme, for example, with a Masters course.

Until recently, clinicians gaining management qualifications were a rarity. Those who did were often focused on using these qualifications as a route to a world beyond medicine, discussed in the final chapter. Over recent years there has been a slow but determined shift, both in the numbers seeking such qualifications and the reasons for wanting to do management courses with increasing numbers of medics gaining qualifications purposefully to remain within the NHS.

A consequence of these trends is that having a management qualification is increasingly seen as a necessity for those competing for success in healthcare. As too often happens in meritocratic environments, whilst initial innovators can succeed with ad hoc experiences, as the group of those with such experiences grows there is an ever-increasing striving for more and often a move towards formalisation. Whereas in the past it may have been sufficient to squeeze in a short course on management in the run up to important job promotion events, the recent trends mean that clinicians are realising that more formal qualifications and often experience are needed to stand out from the crowd. There are many short courses popular with trainees, including those run by The King's Fund and Cumberlege Connections. However, their brevity makes them an entirely different value proposition to an MBA and, therefore, are not considered here in more detail.

In response to the growing demand for management training for medics, two different streams have evolved: first, purpose developed focused courses for healthcare professionals, e.g. masters in healthcare management and or leadership; second, healthcare professionals seeking out existing courses (often high status), e.g. MBAs, EMBAs (Executive MBAs) or Masters in Management. Recently, a third stream has appeared – general management courses adapted for healthcare focus, e.g. MBAs with a focus on healthcare management (*see* Table 2.1).

The arguments put forward by those choosing existing non-healthcare specific qualifications are multiple. Frequently these include the desire to be seen to be able to gain entrance to courses that involve proving the ability to compete with high achievers in other industries. Equally, there is the desire to study with and learn from bright individuals with different but often analogous experiences. Furthermore, this group argues that the fundamentals taught in these courses have been determined over a long period of time and if they are of benefit to other industries, why not healthcare? Some choose these courses because of the institutions that offer them, often business schools, or because of the reputation of individual lecturers.

Those seeking focused qualifications counter that much of what is taught on the general courses is irrelevant to healthcare: what benefit is there for a doctor in spending hours of time and concentrated energy learning how to value companies? Furthermore, the cost of programmes such as MBAs is considerable (*see* Chapter 6). For the private sector, this cost is generally recouped within 5–10 years through salary rises. However, this is less likely to be the case for those in the public sector.

BOX 2.1 The options

General management courses:
- MBA (including EMBA)
- Masters in Management

Specific courses:
- Masters in Finance
- Masters in Public Administration

Healthcare specific courses:
- Masters in Healthcare Leadership/ Management
- Masters in Public Health

Crossover course:
- Healthcare specific MBA

Short courses:
- King's Fund Management Courses

MASTERS IN MANAGEMENT

There is considerable overlap between a Masters in Management and a Masters in Business Administration. Whilst both cover similar ground, MBAs tend to be broader and often incorporate more finance-based courses. MBAs have existed for longer and remain better recognised than Masters in Management. This is reflected in the average price of both courses, with Masters in Management costing generally under £10 000 whereas the average MBA costs more than twice as much. Both groups of Masters can be studied full or part-time or as distance learning.

SPECIFIC MASTERS PROGRAMMES

The breadth of Masters programmes with a specific focus offered by institutions is extraordinary. One institution alone offers 25 courses ranging from marketing to accounting via e-technology. Perhaps the best known of such specialised courses are the Masters in Finance (MFA) and the Masters in Public Policy or Administration (MPP/MPA). The MFA is a widely provided course with topics such as: corporate finance, derivative securities, foundations of finance theory, international finance and macroeconomics and global capital markets. For clinicians, depending on your ultimate career goal, there may be substantial difficulties in relating the world of healthcare to courses primarily focused on private finance.

The MPA or MPP is focused on the public sector. Many topics similar to the MBA are covered but through this lens. Topics therefore include finance, management, economics and policy. This course is highly focused on how the mechanisms of government, both central and locally, are evolving – for example through the use of the Third Sector. Whilst there is considerable overlap between MPP and MPA courses, the fundamental differences are that an MPA is more focused on management and slightly less on the mathematical disciplines such as statistics and economics; whereas the MPP is more focused on policy research and analysis.

MASTERS IN HEALTHCARE MANAGEMENT/LEADERSHIP

All practising doctors are responsible for the use of resources; many will also lead teams or be involved in the supervision of colleagues; and most will work in managed systems, whether in the NHS or in the independent, military, prison or other sectors. Doctors have responsibilities to their patients, employers and those who contract their services. This means that doctors are both managers and are managed.

Management for Doctors (2006)

There has been an explosion in the number of Masters in Healthcare Management in the last 10 years. The total number of courses provided now numbers over 50 and providers range from management departments at universities through to business schools, including collaborations with professional bodies such as the Royal College of Physicians.

The majority of these courses fall under the category of Master of Science (MSc), however a few are MA courses. Most are open to clinicians and non-clinicians, with a few courses targeting specific clinician groups such as the Allied Health Professional Clinical Leadership MSc at the City of London, or the MSc in Medical Leadership run by a collaboration between Birkbeck, London School of Hygiene and Tropical Medicine and the Royal College of Physicians, which is aimed at senior level clinicians. Most are part-time with a significant proportion (around 20%) offered as either full or part-time courses. As with Masters in Management the cost is significantly lower than an MBA (*see* Table 2.1).

All Masters tend to cover similar topics, at least as core subjects – for example organisational behaviour, leadership, quality, change management and human resources. Some however bring in more of the components associated with general management courses, e.g. finance and marketing. Perhaps though, a key difference that is noticeable is that these courses tend to expect students to draw on their current healthcare knowledge extensively. The approach to experience-based learning plays a strong role in the syllabi. For example, the Masters in Medical Leadership at Warwick University is aimed for senior, more experienced doctors. The tuition fees for this taught Master programme is £15 000. It is based around the competency outcomes of the Medical Leadership Competency Framework (Chapter 3) and places value on external speakers and learning from comparative healthcare systems, including an international study trip.

Some universities offer programmes such as these to medical students as an option for third-year studies, i.e. in place of more traditional choices such as Pathology. The response and effect on medical students has been remarkable.

MASTERS IN PUBLIC HEALTH

Masters in Public Health (MPH) forms the backbone of the taught training component of Public Health in the UK. Increasingly, clinicians who practice other specialties of medicine are undertaking these programmes. As with an MBA, the MPH is devised to provide knowledge of topics considered core to public health: epidemiology, biostatistics, environmental health, ethics, social determinants of disease and health service administration (management). Many MPH programmes also have streams that allow a focus on a particular area such as global health, clinical effectiveness, management or quantitative methods.

Both the MBA and the MPH have qualitative and quantitative components, and there is overlap. For example, MPH programmes teach management-related issues such as leadership and change management – albeit within a solely healthcare-related arena in the main. Some MPH programmes do use wider examples, particularly if they are taught in universities with business schools, although this may not extend beyond the case study.

The arguments for doing an MPH above an MBA relate mainly to relevance. Many feel that the breadth of topics covered by an MPH is more relevant for a clinician than those covered by an MBA. In particular, an MPH gives clinicians a strong understanding of how to use evidence-based medicine within clinical practice as well as providing insight into wider healthcare issues. Thus an MPH not only broadens experience and understanding beyond day-to-day clinical medicine, but also enhances the ability to act as a clinician (Box 2.2).

It could, however, be counter-argued that an MBA does enhance the clinical workplace through improving the ability to manage the service, e.g. helping clinicians to understand demand and supply allows them to make sensible and easy to action business cases that span clinical need with financial understanding (*see* Chapter 8).

BOX 2.2 Masters in Public Health

Dr James Mountford, Director of Clinical Quality at UCL Partners

With a background in clinical medicine and management consulting, I chose to do an MPH. I never really considered an MBA. This was a personal decision based on my career aims and circumstances. With equal merit in both – how to choose?

First, some obvious things that both offer: in both you get the 'stamp' of a graduate degree; the knowledge, network and confidence that come with that. Both provide the opportunity for graduate study – one of life's finer gifts.

So how do they differ?

Why an MPH?
First, you need one to be a public health physician, or for PhD-level study in public health. Many MPHs are people with specific career aims in health services research/epidemiology, clinicians looking for training in research methods or people looking to work in government/ international health agencies (an MPH is a very helpful addition to curriculum vitae aimed at WHO, GAVI and similar bodies). MPHs (not surprisingly) offer a grounding in techniques and approaches of public health: epidemiology, biostatistics, social & environmental health, health economics, policy and ethics, among others. (To medics, it's often surprising how different the techniques and ways of thinking are in public health compared to medicine: a population and system focus rather than a patient focus.) You also get access to go deeper in your area of interest: for example, into research methods, developing world health system challenges, social determinants of health or epidemiology. My own focus was health policy and management. For clinicians with research aspirations, an MPH can be a fast way to gain both competence and confidence in research design, methods and statistics.

Why an MBA?

An MBA has the benefits (and the disadvantages) of offering a much more general grounding. The basic axes are usually the functions of management and business, such as finance, accounting, strategy, marketing and operations as well as 'softer' skills like negotiation. Unless your MBA is specifically healthcare focused, there is no need for healthcare to appear on your curriculum at all, though you might *choose* to take courses that focus on health economics, policy and management. Your network will be much broader – with all the benefits for those who intend to pursue careers in healthcare, and the drawbacks of having less deep networks in your chosen field. What you won't get in an MBA is chance for much immersion in the specialist technical skills used in careers in and around public health or clinical research.

Only you can make the decision. If you see your career as heading primarily into healthcare management, you have a real choice – an MBA might be a better fit (and better regarded), but consider a management-focused MPH. If you want technical health research skills, do an MPH. Whichever you do, if your school allows it, look for opportunities to take courses outside your 'home' school: possibly in a School of Public Policy . . . maybe it is an MPA you should be doing?

HEALTHCARE-SPECIFIC MBA

Few business schools have started to provide MBAs with a healthcare focus. These tend to maintain the MBA base and orientate toward healthcare. The most well-established of these is the MBA (Health Executive) run by Keele University. This comprises six one-week courses over two years including:

➤ Health Policy and Strategy
➤ Health Economics
➤ Human Resource Management
➤ Management Science
➤ Accounting and Financial Management
➤ Operations Management.

As with business-focused MBAs, these core modules are followed by a personal research dissertation (approximately 20 000 words) undertaken over 9/12 months. Without the dissertation, completion of the above modules qualifies participants for a Diploma. Unlike most business school MBAs, assessment for the Keele MBA (Health Executive) is 100 per cent based on assignments rather than formal examinations. The student profile at Keele is a fairly even three-way split between doctors at various levels of training, from junior specialty trainees through to consultants; other health professionals including nurses, podiatrists and physiotherapists – usually with some management experience or responsibility; and health service managers from a variety of backgrounds.

A further iteration of this programme is collaboration between the Open University and the *British Medical Journal* (*BMJ*). Like Keele, this modular system setup allows individuals to accrue credits that can lead to a healthcare-focused MBA. Other MBA programmes generally offer electives that relate specifically to healthcare.

Whilst it may seem that healthcare MBAs provide the ideal meshing together of healthcare and business, these courses are relatively new and currently few people outside the institutions teaching have a strong understanding of the concept. Thus for those contemplating this option, the balance between course reputation and relevance is important to weigh up.

MANAGEMENT VALIDATION

If the purpose of undertaking an MBA is to demonstrate management expertise, an alternative approach to the above Masters is to consider the range of qualifications offered by the Chartered Management Institute, described in Box 2.3. NHS managers and the military are more familiar with this option, which is modular in approach and involves submitting a portfolio annually.

BOX 2.3 Chartered Management Institute

Dr Edward Nicol MD MRCP

Whilst MBAs remain a mainstay of academic managerial and business knowledge, there are alternative mechanisms to explore managerial leadership via a more mixed vocational and practical route. It is possible to gain a certificate, diploma or executive diploma in management in a step-wise manner prior to, or instead of, an MBA, and this may allow individuals to tailor their managerial journey to their developing professional role. These attract credits towards an MBA should participants wish to pursue this at a later date.

The Chartered Management Institute (CMI) offers, in addition to the qualifications described above, the vocational Chartered Manager designation (CMgr). This involves a vocational-based assessment that requires demonstration of real-life managerial competence and good practice. Whilst Diplomas and Masters Degrees denote academic understanding the CMgr designation denotes demonstration of a real practical experience and learning and is widely respected in managerial circles. In addition, the Chartered Management Institute, like the Royal Medical Colleges, offer membership, fellowship and companionship levels of involvement, again offered based on practical experience and expertise.

Membership at all levels provides many benefits including both CPD and access to a wide network of managers, both regionally and nationally, from all sectors.

SUMMARY

The decision to commence any Masters degree is a challenging one. The work entailed in studying for such a degree is considerable. An MBA is an opportunity to explore a world that is unfamiliar to clinicians, and whilst that is attractive to many, it does reduce the direct relevance to healthcare.

There is a wide range of alternatives to MBAs, summarised in Table 2.1. These overlap to varying degrees with an MBA. Some are more healthcare-focused, others are less so.

There is no best option. Key to making the right decision is knowledge of the

TABLE 2.1 Comparison between MBA and other related courses

Category	Masters in Management	Specific Masters programmes	Masters in Healthcare Management/Leadership	Masters in Public Health	Healthcare specific MBA
Content	Similar content to MBA but often less focus on finance and more focus on organisational issues, such as change management.	Limited overlap with MBA – a feature of MBA may be drawn out in detail, e.g. marketing/finance.	Focus tends to be less on finance than an MBA. Similar in content to a Masters in Management but with a healthcare slant, e.g. focus on current healthcare policies.	As with an MBA, an MPH provides a general overview of the topic, i.e. public health, thus incorporating aspects of an MBA, e.g. management.	Consistent with MBA but with the addition of healthcare-related options.
Recognition	Less recognised currently.	Particularly the MFA and MPP/PA are well recognised.	Less recognised than an MBA but increasingly renowned particularly as collaborations grow between key medical bodies and universities.	Well recognised within healthcare circles, less so beyond. Recognition does not necessarily link to the managerial aspects however.	Less established than classic generalist MBA. Few of the top 10 FT ranked schools offer such a tailored programme.
Cost	Courses tend to be considerably cheaper than MBAs, often costing a quarter to a half of a traditional UK MBA programme.	Cost is lower than an MBA although MPP/ MPA more expensive than general management courses.	Cost is lower than an MBA and more in line with a Masters in Management.	More equivalent to a specialised general course, thus less than an MBA in the main.	In line with MBA.

options. Some individuals even decide that a combination of courses is the best solution, e.g. an MPH and an MBA. Understanding the variety of courses available and their nuances is fundamental, as is understanding what motivates the said individual seeking such an option.

All programmes can be viewed on websites (*see* Further reading). Many provide brochures and open evenings. Most will happily link prospective students to existing or past students. As more clinicians take part in these programmes, knowledge about the individual courses will become both more accessible and more mainstream.

FURTHER READING

Bradford University School of Management. The Bradford MSc. www.bradford.ac.uk/management/programmes/msc/

Cass Business School, University of London. www.cass.city.ac.uk/

Chartered Management Institute. Qualifications. Available at: www2.managers.org.uk/The_Hub_Menu_1.aspx?id=10:5176

EMYLON Business School. European Master in Management. www.em-lyon.com/english/grad/emm/index.aspx

ESCP. ESCP Europe Master in Management. www.escpeurope.eu/escp-europe-programmes/master-in-management/welcome-to-the-escp-europe-master-in-management/

Financial Times. Business school rankings. www.ft.com/businesseducation/mba

Ham C, Clark J, Spurgeon P, *et al.* (2010). *Medical Chief Executives in the NHS: facilitators and barriers to their career progress.* London: NHS Institute for Innovation and Improvement and Academy of Medical Royal Colleges.

Imperial College Business School, London. MSc Management. www3.imperial.ac.uk/business-school/programmes/msc-management

LSE Management. Masters in Management. www.lse.ac.uk/collections/management/MastersinManagement.htm

Manchester Business School, University of Manchester. Specialist Masters. www.mbs.ac.uk/specialist/index.aspx

Mintzberg H (2004). *Managers Not MBAs: a hard look at the soft practice of managing and management development.* San Francisco, CA: Berrett-Koehler Publishers, Inc.

Saïd Business School and NHS (2009–2012). *Increasing the Motivation and Ability of Health Care Managers to Access and Use Management Research. SDO Project – 08/1808/242.* Summary available at: www.sdo.nihr.ac.uk/projdetails.php?ref=08-1808-242 (accessed 18 June 2010).

University of Bath, School of Management. MSc programmes. www.bath.ac.uk/management/courses/msc/

University of Strathclyde Business School. Management. www.strath.ac.uk/management/

CHAPTER 3

How does an MBA fit with current health policy?

Clinical leadership is putting clinicians at the heart of shaping and running clinical services, so as to deliver excellent outcomes for patients and populations, not as a one-off task or project, but as a core part of clinicians' professional identity.

James Mountford, Director of Quality, UCL Partners

INTRODUCTION

With the prolific industry of courses, qualifications and secondments in clinical leadership, outlined in Chapter 2, this chapter provides an overview of where an MBA relates to current health policy.

The General Medical Council (GMC) describes leadership as key to doctors' professional work and 'vital' that doctors contribute towards the effective running of organisations in which they work, influencing their future direction. Perhaps even moreso with the shift to GP consortia commissioning of healthcare.

Relevant to doctors' professional work are the seven principles of conduct for holders of public office: selflessness, integrity, objectivity, accountability, openness, honesty and leadership. These were originally set out by the Nolan committee, now the Committee on Standards in Public Life, established as an independent committee in 1994.

NEXT STAGE REVIEW (NSR)

In 2007, then Prime Minister Gordon Brown created a 'Government of All Talents' (GOATs). For better or for worse, this included appointing and ennobling former CBI Chief Sir Digby Jones, top surgeon Ara Darzi, ex-UN Deputy Secretary General Mark Malloch Brown and former First Sea Lord Admiral Sir Alan West, amongst others. By 2009, few GOATs remained, but the legacy of Professor the Lord Ara Darzi of Denham's Ministerial interlude will be best remembered for the Next Stage Review (NSR) (DH, 2008). This review marked the 60-year anniversary of the NHS and aimed to renew the NHS for the twenty-first century.

Over 2000 health and social care professionals reviewed the best evidence available and discussed healthcare priorities. In addition, both patients and the public contributed to the NSR. Relevant to this book, the review concluded:

> Greater freedom, enhanced accountability and empowering staff are necessary but not sufficient in the pursuit of high quality care. Making change actually happen takes leadership. It is central to our expectations of the healthcare professionals of tomorrow.

Quality care is explained succinctly by three measurable and memorable dimensions: patient safety; patient experience and effectiveness of care. The core job of healthcare professionals is to provide high quality care for patients. Safety is a core component to providing high quality healthcare. The three dimensions of quality above are adapted from the Institute of Medicine's seminal report (2001), which identifies the following six dimensions of quality in healthcare:

1 **Safe**: avoid injuries to patients from care that is intended to help them.
2 **Effective**: provide services based on scientific knowledge to all who could benefit, and refrain from providing services to those not likely to benefit.
3 **Patient-centred**: provide care that is respectful of and responsive to individual patient preferences, needs and values, and ensure that patient values guide all clinical decisions.
4 **Timely**: reduce waits for both those who receive and those who give care.
5 **Effective**: avoid waste of equipment, supplies, ideas and energy.
6 **Equitable**: provide care that does not vary in quality because of personal characteristics such as gender, ethnicity, geographic location and socioeconomic status.

The NSR compared the NHS to large American healthcare organisations, such as Kaiser Permanente, and identified the NHS as an organisation with relatively few clinicians in leadership roles. This is despite a growing parallel body of literature on 'new professionalism' identifying the potential wider role of the clinician as practitioner, partner and leader. However, it is unrealistic to expect clinicians to take on leadership roles without making it integral to their training and development. The NSR identified several mechanisms to make this rhetoric a reality, increasing the supply of clinical leaders. One of these recommendations is the National Leadership Council (NLC), chaired by the NHS Chief Executive, responsible for overseeing all matters of leadership across healthcare.

MEDICAL LEADERSHIP COMPETENCY FRAMEWORK (MLCF)

At the same time as the NSR was underway, the Academy of Medical Royal Colleges and the NHS Institute for Innovation and Improvement jointly developed the MLCF, following consultation with a wide range of stakeholders. The MLCF maps out the leadership competencies that doctors need to become more actively involved in the planning, delivery and transformation of services for patients – the vision set out in the NSR. The MLCF was originally published in May 2008 and is updated annually. This framework is designed to be relevant to all stages of training and is not restricted to those in formal leadership roles. The MLCF model of shared leadership emphasises teamwork rather than individual performance. To date, no other healthcare system has systematically reviewed and developed a comparable leadership framework.

The MLCF aims to meet the challenge articulated by Professor John Tooke, *Aspiring to Excellence* (2008):

> The doctor's frequent role as head of the healthcare team and commander of considerable clinical resource requires that greater attention is paid to management and leadership skills regardless of specialism. An acknowledgement of the leadership role of medicine is increasingly evident. Role acknowledgement and aspiration to enhanced roles be they in subspecialty practice, management and leadership, education or research are likely to facilitate greater clinical engagement.

There are five core areas of competence in the MLCF, as shown in Table 3.1. Each

TABLE 3.1 Medical Leadership Competency Framework

Developing personal qualities	Developing self-awareness
	Managing yourself
	Continuing personal development
	Acting with integrity
Working with others	Developing networks
	Building and maintaining relationships
	Encouraging contribution
	Working within teams
Managing services	Planning
	Managing resources
	Managing people
	Managing performance
Improving services	Ensuring patient safety
	Critically evaluating
	Encouraging improvement and innovation
	Facilitating transformation
Setting direction	Identifying the contexts for change
	Applying knowledge and evidence
	Making decisions
	Evaluating impact

Reproduced with permission from Academy of Royal Colleges and NHS Institute for Innovation and Improvement (2009). *Medical Leadership Competency Framework*. 2nd ed. Coventry: NHS Institute for Innovation and Improvement.

of these areas overlaps with the MBA syllabus in Section 3 of this book. The MLCF is applied to three distinct career stages. Stage 1 is up to the end of undergraduate training. This is mainly about demonstrating personal qualities and working with others. There are fewer opportunities for undergraduates to be involved in the other domains, particularly setting direction. Stage 2 is for specialty training, up to the end of postgraduate training. Stage 3 is for consultants and GPs, post-specialist certification, where all leadership competencies apply.

The MLCF has recently been developed into the generic Clinical Leadership Competency Framework with the NLC, as described below.

NATIONAL LEADERSHIP COUNCIL

As described in the NSR, the National Leadership Council (NLC) is a sub-committee of the NHS Management Board, chaired by the NHS Chief Executive. It was created in April 2009 with the vision to create a 'NHS with outstanding leadership and leadership development at every level to ensure high quality care for all'. The current focus of the council is on five work streams: clinical leadership, board development, top leaders, emerging leaders and inclusion. The reason for a specific focus on clinical leadership is because of the below barriers to clinicians entering leadership positions. These are genuine risks for medics with MBAs to be aware of and consider:
➤ potential risk of loss of status and formal registration to practice
➤ impact on future revalidation
➤ contractural issues for re-entry into clinical role
➤ vulnerability as a manager to job loss
➤ exposure to adverse media comment at the highest level.

The clinical leadership work stream of the NLC focuses on new roles for clinicians, challenging the historic prejudices within the system that have led to the above barriers. It maps accreditation for organisations delivering leadership across to the work of quality assurance for NHS managers. The NLC aims to ensure that clinicians are introduced to leadership at the start of their professional training, recognising that while not everyone is a leader, everyone is able to improve services:

> Leadership is for the whole NHS, not just for those in management roles. Clinicians with leadership skills have the greatest ability to deliver better services for patients and foster innovation, quality and safety.

To achieve this, the NLC has provided funding for Leadership Fellowships for all healthcare professionals, not solely doctors. In addition, the Emerging Leaders work stream of the NLC brings together healthcare professionals from a wide range of backgrounds to stimulate interprofessional learning and development. These are aligned to the QIPP agenda (Quality, Innovation, Productivity and Prevention) and are complimentary to the pre-existing fellowships such as Darzi Fellows. Of note, for academically orientated medics with MBAs, future NLC funding has also been allocated for future professors of Clinical Leadership in universities.

SUMMARY

This chapter has summarised the relevance of the NSR, MLCF and the Clinical Leadership workstream of the NLC specifically for doctors interested in leadership and considering doing an MBA. The final two chapters of this book consider the longer-term career opportunities for medics with MBAs, relative to the policy initiatives presented here.

FURTHER READING

Committee on Standards in Public Life (2010). *Annual Review and Report 2008–2009*. London: Committee on Standards in Public Life.

Department of Health (2008). *Next Stage Review*. London: Department of Health.

Department of Health (2010). *Clinical Leadership: interim report*. London: National Leadership Council.

General Medical Council (2003, 2009). *Tomorrow's Doctors*. London: GMC.

General Medical Council (2006). *Management for Doctors*. London: GMC.

Ham C, Clark J, Spurgeon P, *et al.* (2010). *Medical Chief Executives in the NHS: facilitators and barriers to their career progress*. Academy of Medical Royal Colleges, University of Warwick, NHS Institute for Innovation and Improvement, University of Birmingham.

Institute of Medicine (2001). *Crossing the Quality Chasm: a new health system for the 21st century*. Washington, DC: National Academy Press.

National Leadership Council (2010). *Clinical Leadership Interim Report*. London: NHS.

NHS Institute for Innovation and Improvement. www.institute.nhs.uk

NHS Institute for Innovation and Improvement, Academy of Medical Royal Colleges (2008). *Medical Leadership Competency Framework*. 2nd ed. Coventry: NHS Institute for Innovation and Improvement.

Tooke J (2008). *Aspiring to Excellence: independent inquiry into modernising medical careers*. London: Department of Health.

SECTION 2

How to do an MBA?

Innovation has become a 'buzzword' in healthcare. There is much that healthcare could learn from other industries about managing innovation. In his book, *Dealing with Darwin*, Moore dispels three myths below about innovation, for healthcare professionals to take heed:

➤ Innovation in and of itself is valuable.
➤ Innovation becomes less necessary and less possible as categories mature.
➤ The essence of innovation is the same in any company.

Healthcare is under increasing pressure to innovate to provide sufficient care to meet the needs of an ageing demographic within budget restrictions. Thus individual healthcare professionals feel under pressure to be innovative in their approach. As described by Moore, innovation is only of value if it helps to achieve economic advantage. Unless innovation is managed, it is possible that it only serves to create more waste.

Securing an MBA as a medic is an innovative career path that can be achieved through a variety of means, discussed in the following section of this book. There are opportunities to think innovatively about where and how to study, as well as sources of funding. However, it is not in the doing of an MBA that value is created. Value lies in what you do with it thereafter.

FURTHER READING

Moore G (2005). *Dealing with Darwin: how great companies innovate at every phase of their evolution*. New York: Penguin.

CHAPTER 4

The logistics of planning an MBA

Trust yourself. You know more than you think you do.

Benjamin Spock, paediatrician

INTRODUCTION

Preceding chapters have made the case for MBAs in healthcare and the corporate sector as well as examining alternative qualifications. This chapter will consider how to choose the right MBA for each individual. This chapter is designed to provide a framework for how to think about the various options, and to allow potential students to make informed choices.

WHEN TO DO AN MBA?

For many doctors, the realisation that a further degree with a management flavour is of interest to them develops from an event, or series of events, related to clinical practice. It may be frustration at trying to institute changes and not having the language or knowledge to convince those that hold the purse strings, or it may be a feeling of floundering as seniority brings additional managerial responsibilities. Increasingly, these thoughts are generated early in a medical career and are preambles to decisions about alternative careers within healthcare, such as eventual roles as Medical Director or CEO, discussed in Section 4.

There is no one moment most fitting to do an MBA. Rather that situation and circumstance align at different points for different people. There are perhaps moments in medical training when it is harder to fulfil the obligations of an MBA, e.g. alongside royal college membership exams, or just pre-job applications. However, this too very much depends on the individual. Similarly, the type of MBA chosen, e.g. part-time or full-time, plays into the timing versus career progression debate. For those keen on taking a year out of training it can be easier to do so at certain points, e.g. between the key break points like Foundation to Specialty Training (as in Box 4.2). Although some may argue that for doctors in training it is less intimidating to take time out as they have the luxury of knowing that a protected job awaits, this very much depends on the flexibility of the local Deanery and employing Trust. For more senior doctors it may be that sabbatical years could be used for the purpose of achieving an MBA.

Doing the MBA as an executive programme mitigates the need for some of the decision-making, as time does not necessarily need to be taken from day-to-day work. Although, some programmes require weekday attendance, that would be difficult to manage with current study leave entitlement alone. The hours of work around set teaching are not inconsiderable and need to be factored into the decision-making process outlined in Box 4.1.

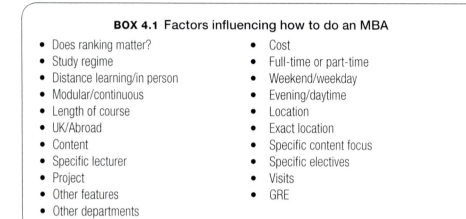

BOX 4.1 Factors influencing how to do an MBA

- Does ranking matter?
- Study regime
- Distance learning/in person
- Modular/continuous
- Length of course
- UK/Abroad
- Content
- Specific lecturer
- Project
- Other features
- Other departments

- Cost
- Full-time or part-time
- Weekend/weekday
- Evening/daytime
- Location
- Exact location
- Specific content focus
- Specific electives
- Visits
- GRE

Choosing an MBA can feel a bit like a rubix cube: once you have one bit lined up the others fall out of place. Key to the decision-making is continually analysing your priorities: does cost outweigh reputation or does the course content outweigh the location? For many, these choices are pre-determined, constrained by external factors like housing or family; for others each needs careful thought. Each of the domains outlined in the box above are intrinsically interwoven with each other: location is bound up with reputation and cost; study regime relates to ranking and content. Thus each domain needs to be examined and the domains ranked by individuals according to personal priorities. Dr Graham Rich, Medical Chief Executive, describes his thought processes for doing an MBA in Box 4.2.

BOX 4.2 Dr Graham Rich, Former CEO of University Hospitals Bristol NHS Foundation Trust

For Dr Rich the timing was clear: 'I had completed GP training and got all my exams, and it was a natural break'.

Similarly, Dr Rich chose his MBA course because: 'A friend of mine was doing a MBA at London Business School at the time and advised me to go for an institution with a high reputation given that so many universities offer MBAs. He recommended INSEAD, LBS, IMD, Warwick and Manchester. I was not interested in the business schools in the USA because they take two years and I couldn't afford the time or the money. I had worked out that if I got a Rotary Foundation scholarship they would pay my fees and some living expenses at an overseas institution, but not in the UK. That narrowed the field down to INSEAD and IMD. I chose INSEAD, because it had a slightly younger age profile, was more international and more taught in English. Plus INSEAD had a well developed and strong alumni network. And I had heard that they have great parties. So the choice was easy'.

Dr Rich's decision-making was very much influenced by funding options: 'It was funded by a Rotary Foundation scholarship plus some debt. I remain eternally grateful to the Rotary Club for selecting me for this competitive fellowship. They fund a few non-rotarians to study abroad each year. It also meant that I visited some French and English Rotary Clubs and spoke about my experiences'.

For him, the choice of full-time vs. part-time was clear: 'I think part-time MBAs are very difficult to manage, particularly if you have a family as well as a job. I applaud anyone who can manage their time so well. I think 50% of the learning comes from interaction with other participants and so if you choose a distance learning MBA you miss out on this aspect, although several programmes get participants together for short periods to compensate for this'.

As are the benefits to all: 'A more integrated approach to management and clinical thinking is to be welcomed. Even if clinicians don't become service leaders or managers, the MBA would help them understand systems, negotiate with confidence, etc. Hopefully more doctors will seek to embrace an early role in leadership and management'.

DOES RANKING MATTER?

Perhaps the easiest place to start is to consider how much reputation matters. For individuals outside healthcare, having an MBA is often not enough. Having an MBA from a top business school is key, partly because of the kudos this brings and partly because of the networks created. In healthcare, it is currently still unusual to possess an MBA and so perhaps this is less important.

If reputation matters, a good starting point is perusing rankings such as the *Financial Times* Ranking. This will give a flavour of which are the top business schools. The *Financial Times* rankings are split into executive programmes and full-time programmes, Tables 4.1 and 4.2. It is important to remember that this ranking, along with many others, has specific criteria on which it judges business schools and these may not equate to an individual's preference structure. For example, the FT takes into account salary increase post MBA. For a public sector worker this may be less relevant.

Issues around the cost and funding of MBAs are discussed in the following chapter.

STUDY REGIME

Perhaps the next question to consider is the logistics of the programme. The first of these questions surrounds taking the MBA full-time or part-time. Full-time courses allow individuals the opportunity to immerse themselves in the business school: the MBA becomes the students' world for the duration of the course. This has advantages: many students become highly active in the groups and networks that business schools seed. It allows individuals to attend additional events, lectures and dragons den experiences. It creates the informal time for planning and developing new ideas, and constructive discussion. Doing a full-time course means less conflicting demands on time, with no shifts or clinics at precisely the moment that a crucial essay or exam is due. Full-time also means that there are extended holiday periods in which to take part in placements and to hone CVs (business CVs are notoriously shorter and sharper than lengthy medical CVs). In addition, doing a full-time MBA means not earning a salary for at least one year and this is often the deciding factor for many. Whilst it is sometimes feasible to take some time out of clinical practice, this may not always be possible due to training or staffing requirements.

Equally there are disadvantages. As described in Chapter 1, those doing full-time courses tend to be younger and so the networking opportunities may be less mature, taking time to become useful as individuals grow into new and exciting roles. Similarly, the experience that students bring to class discussions and group work is often more limited, as a result of more restricted world experience. Whilst grappling with the dual demands of a job and a Masters are challenging, it can be useful to have ongoing experiences which add relevance to the taught experience. For project work, it is sometimes easier to gain access to data and people if they are connected to your day-to-day role.

Having made the decision about whether full- or part-time is preferable; there are a series of further decisions, especially if the part-time option is being explored. First, executive (part-time) programmes are available in a number of different formats. The most extreme choices within executive programmes are between distance and in-person programmes. For many, the ability to work at one's own pace, in the comfort of one's own surroundings, through web based learning is ideal (*see* Case Study in Chapter 16). These programmes provide great flexibility in terms of the time commitment and duration of the programme. Furthermore, many also allow participants to take part in some face-to-face learning.

Whilst the flexibility is important for many, the cost of this is the loss of interaction with other students, the networking opportunities, the dedicated time to work on the material (it is often harder to carve out time when in the home environment) and the benefit of interactive teaching including lectures and small groups.

An important consideration when deciding therefore on whether distance learning is the best approach, is of the learning style that best suits the individual. It may be that a teaching system dependent on self-motivation and focus is the modality of choice. Alternatively, one where stimulation and enthusiasm is shared may be preferable.

If the decision is that in-person learning is the modality of choice, then a further sub-set of options needs to be considered. First, as already discussed in the section on timing, does the applicant have the luxury of sufficient weekday time or will the course need to be primarily weekend-based? Executive programmes exist in both categories although most weekend courses include a Friday. Similarly, there are executive programmes that are evening focused rather than daytime.

A second sub-option is whether the course need be modular or continuous. For many, having discrete blocks is preferable to sacrificing every weekend for 18 months. Although for those with childcare, to arrange the routine engendered by the latter option may be preferable.

Each of these sub-options also feeds into thinking about whether the duration of the course matters. Full-time courses range from one year in Europe to two in the

USA. Part-time programmes can be short (around 18 months) or extend for many years. Thus part of the self-analysis needs to be around how this fits with other life choices, including stage of career.

An important additional aspect to this is that all too often, doing a Masters programme and working can lead to a sensation of 'having something hanging over you', such that there is a constant niggle. Holidays end up planned around essays or exams, with heavy text books carted around the world. Time is often spent worrying about how to juggle commitments. All in all, the time spent on an MBA can be a time of great personal struggle as well as triumph. It is important to think about for how long this is sustainable and whether it is preferable to have short sharp bursts of frenzied activity or a more drawn out experience.

LOCATION

Alongside thinking about the study regime are decisions around the geographic location of the course. As with all factors previously discussed, location is intrinsically bound up with the others. For example, if ranking is your key domain then it may be that courses outside the UK are worth investigating, or an executive programme that has a UK and 'other' component would suffice. Tables 4.1 and 4.2 show that many of the top ranked courses are non-UK based.

Perhaps though, the starting point here needs to be thought around the country or countries that are important for the participant. It may be that personal, financial or other constraints rule out foreign travel. Or it may be that part of the desire to do an MBA is to have a different experience including living in a different country. If non-UK countries are considered then it is worth bearing in mind the language requirements of individual courses.

Increasingly, executive programmes are linked across multiple countries, some criss-cross developed and developing world economies. For example, Columbia University and LBS run a highly ranked Executive MBA (EMBA) programme.

Choosing a UK course does not rule out developing an understanding of other countries' business models. Many courses include options to look at individual countries or groups of countries, e.g. Business in China courses. Similarly, increasing numbers of courses (both full-time and part-time) offer electives based in other countries, e.g. study tours to China. These often consist of a combination of lectures and visits to key businesses and provide an opportunity to see part of the world that is hard to gain admittance too as an individual.

Within the UK, geography may also be a factor that is of high importance to applicants. The time commitment demanded by an MBA is considerable and many would perhaps wisely wonder at the sense of spending additional hours commuting to distant locations for the course. Yet, many do this both on full-time and executive courses, with many participants to UK courses coming from places as distant as Australia or China. Thus, settling for a UK course does not per se mean that the networks created will be less international.

CONTENT

In many ways, a sub component of rankings or reputation that may be important is the strength or indeed existence of a department that is interested in healthcare. Some, for example Harvard, Saïd and Imperial, have or are building strong healthcare faculties and it may be important to the applicant that this is present.

For others, this may matter less as part of the point of doing an MBA is to escape from the confines of the health or indeed public sector. Thus it may be a course element other than healthcare that is the draw. Some courses focus on entrepreneurship, others more on finance or strategy and it might be this that helps crystallise the decision-making.

Some go as far as to choose MBA programmes because of specific lecturers – big draw names like Michael Porter at Harvard have strong attraction. However, there is always the risk that these individuals will not teach their usual courses the particular year the applicant attends.

As already hinted, the opportunity to pursue certain elective choices, type of project or visit can be a deciding factor in MBA choices. However, it is important to bear in mind the risk that courses do not run in a given year because of dependence on individual lecturer skills or re-fashioning of departments and/or curricula.

One final factor that may impact on decision-making is the quality of other departments at the university, as it is sometimes possible to gain credits from these departments as part of the MBA. Thus it might be the presence of a school of public health that clinches the decision-making.

SUMMARY

This chapter provides a framework (Box 4.1) to use in thinking about when, where and how to do an MBA. It cannot provide prescriptive answers, more serves to act as a guide for considered self-reflection about individual priorities.

An MBA is such a considerable financial and time commitment that examining all the options is the best way to ensure that the eventual choice made allows the individual the best chance of success and enjoyment of the experience.

TABLE 4.1 Top UK full-time MBA programmes as ranked by the *Financial Times* (2010)

Institution	Ranking in 2010	Cost	Study regime Full- or Part-time	Length of course	Location UK or abroad	Exact location	Other GMAT required	Work experience	Academic criteria	Application process	Ability to take credits elsewhere
LBS	1	49 900	Full	15–21 months	UK	London	Yes	More than 3 years preferred	Good degree preferable	Essays and interview	Yes
Oxford-Saïd	16	36 000	Full	12 months	UK	Oxford	Yes average 680	More than 3 years preferred	2:1 or above as a guide	Essays and interview	
Cambridge-Judge	21	35 000 + average of 2249 college fee	Full	12 months	UK	Cambridge	Yes with specifics	3 years minimum	2:1 or above	Essays and interview	
Lancaster	24	23 500	Full	12 months	UK	Lancaster	Yes more than 600	3 years minimum	Honours degree or equivalent	Essays and interview	
Cranfield	26	31 000	Full	12 months	UK	Cranfield	Balanced GMAT score	More than 3 years preferred	Good degree	Essays and interview	Cranfield
Imperial	32	34 000	Full	12 months	UK	London	Yes more than 600	3 years minimum	Good degree	Essays and interview	Imperial
Manchester	40	34 400	Full	12 months	UK	Manchester	Balanced GMAT score	Usually 3 years minimum	Good degree	Essays and interview	
City University: Cass	41	31 000	Full	12 months	UK	London	Yes more than 640	3 years minimum	Good degree	Essays and interview	City University: Cass
Warwick	42	21 400	Full	12 months	UK	Warwick	Balanced GMAT score	3 years minimum	Good degree	Essays and interview	
Strathclyde	51	21 000	Full	12 months	UK	Strathclyde	No	3 years minimum and be over 24 years old	Good degree or professional qualification	Essays and interview	

NB Application fees extra.
NB US equivalent to UK degrees accepted. e.g. GPA 3.5 or higher.

TABLE 4.2 Top UK Executive MBA programmes as ranked by the *Financial Times* (2009)

Institution	Ranking in 2009	Cost	Study regime					Length of course	Location		Other		Academic criteria	Application process
			Full- or part-time	Distance learning or in person	Weekend or weekday	Modular or continuous	Evening or daytime		UK or abroad	Exact location	GMAT required	Work experience		
Trium HEC, LSE, NYU	2	80000**	Part-time	In person	Weekday	Modular	Daytime	16 months	UK/US/France	London/New York/Paris	Yes or GRE	Minimum 10 years	–	Initially resume and academic background
EMBA Global Americas and Europe (LBS and Columbia)	3	86000**	Part-time	In person	Mixed	Modular	Daytime	18 months	UK and US	London and New York	Yes	Expected to be considerable	Good degree or alternative	Essays and interview
University of Chicago: Booth	4	69000	Part-time	In person	Mixed	Modular	Daytime	21 months	UK/US/Singapore		No	Strong experience	Good academic background	Essay and interview
LBS	8	53000*	Part-time	In person	Weekend (Friday and Saturday of alternate weeks) at least for first year	Continuous	Daytime	20 months	UK	London	Yes	Typically 5 years and be a 'decision maker'	Good degree or alternative	Essays and interview

Institution	Ranking in 2009	Cost	Study regime						Location	Other			
City University: Cass Weekday	21	42000	Part-time	In person	Weekday	Continuous	Evening – twice a week approx 3 hours	24 months	UK	London	Yes more than 600	Minimum 3 years	Good degree	Essays and interview
City University: Cass Weekend	21	42000	Part-time	In person	Weekend	Continuous	Long weekend Friday to Monday	24 months	UK	London	Yes more than 600	Minimum 3 years	Good degree	Essays and interview
ESCP	25	37000**	Part-time	In person	Weekday	Modular	Daytime	18 months	UK (electives can be done elsewhere)	London	No	Minimum 5 years	Good degree	Essays and interview
Imperial Executive Weekday	31	35500	Part-time	In person	Weekday – every other Friday plus 8 3-day blocks for first year – second year between 17 and 25 weekdays (if 17 then 8 weekend days required)	Continuous	Daytime	24 months	UK	London	No	Minimum 3 years	Good degree or alternative professional qualification	Essays and interview

(continued)

TABLE 4.2 (cont.)

Institution	Ranking in 2009	Cost	Study regime			Location		Other			
Imperial Executive Weekend	31	39 500	Part-time	In person	Weekend – one long weekend a month approx for first year, between 17 and 25 weekdays for second year (if 17 then 8 weekend days required)	Continuous	Daytime	21 months	UK	London	No	Minimum 3 years	Good degree or alternative professional qualification	Essays and interview
Imperial Distance Learning	31	24 035	Part-time	Distance learning	N/A	Continuous	N/A	Approx 3 years depending on choice of elective modules and project	N/A	N/A	GMAT more than 600	Minimum 3 years or good professional qualification	Good degree	Essay and telephone interview
Cranfield Part Time	33	31 000***	Part-time	In person	Mixed (15 weekends Friday – Saturday plus 3 one week modules per year)	Continuous	Daytime	2 years	UK	Cranfield	Balanced GMAT	Minimum 3 years	Good degree	Essay and interview

Institution	Ranking in 2009	Cost	Study regime						Location		Other				
Cranfield Modular	33	31 000***	Part-time	In person	6 8-day residential blocks	Modular	Daytime	2 years	UK	Cranfield	Balanced GMAT	Minimum 3 years	Good degree	Essay and interview
Warwick Part Time	34	24 000^	Part-time	In person	Weekday	Modular	Daytime	Approx 3 years depending on choice of elective modules	UK	Warwick	GMAT may be required	Minimum 4 years	Good degree	Essay and probably interview
Warwick Distance Learning	34	15 600^	Part-time	Distance learning but compulsory 8 day module each September	N/A	Continuous	N/A	Approx 3 years depending on choice of elective modules	N/A	N/A	GMAT may be required	Minimum 4 years	Good degree	Essay and probably interview
Henley	44	39 950	Part-time	In person	Mixed	Modular	Daytime	2 years	UK	Henley	No	Minimum 3 years	Good degree	Essay and ideally selection day

* Includes course text books, hotel for international module, hotel for residential leadership module, student association subscription but not hotel, etc. for second optional international module.

** Based on exchange rate January 2010.

*** Includes most of the costs of international elective and laptop for use during course.

^ Fees are 8000 for the first year and then rise according to university increases from this baseline p.a., with additional costs for electives/extension.

NB variation between courses as to whether text books are covered, etc.

NB Application fees extra.

NB US equivalent to UK degrees accepted, e.g. GPA 3.5 or higher.

FURTHER READING

Cass Business School, City University London. www.cass.city.ac.uk/

Cass Business School, City University London. Executive MBA. www.cass.city.ac.uk/mba/emba/index.html

Chicago Booth. Executive MBA programme. www.chicagobooth.edu/ExecMBA/

Cranfield University, School of Management. www.som.cranfield.ac.uk/som/

ESCP Europe. European Executive MBA. www.escpeurope.eu/nc/escp-europe-programmes/european-executive-mba/european-executive-mba-programme-overview-escp-europe/

Financial Times. About the FT business school rankings. http://rankings.ft.com/businessschoolrankings/

Henley University of Reading. The Henley Executive MBA. www.henley.reading.ac.uk/management/mba/mgmt-executivemodularmba.aspx

Imperial College London. Imperial Executive MBA. www3.imperial.ac.uk/business-school/programmes/executive-mba

Imperial College London. Imperial MBA. www3.imperial.ac.uk/business-school/programmes/imperial-mba

INSEAD. www.insead.edu

Judge Business School, Cambridge University. The Cambridge MBA. www.jbs.cam.ac.uk/mba/

Lancaster University Management School. The Lancaster full-time MBA. www.lums.lancs.ac.uk/masters/mba/

London Business School. Executive MBA. www.london.edu/programmes/executivemba.html

London Business School, Columbia Business School. EMBA-Global. www.emba-global.com/

London Business School. MBA. www.london.edu/programmes/mba.html

Manchester Business School, University of Manchester. www.mbs.ac.uk/

Saïd Business School, University of Oxford. www.sbs.ox.ac.uk/Pages/default.aspx

Trium Global Executive MBA. www.triumemba.org/

University of Strathclyde Business School. The Strathclyde MBA. www.strath.ac.uk/management/mba/

Warwick Business School. The Warwick MBA. www.wbs.ac.uk/students/mba/

CHAPTER 5

Money matters

If you think education is expensive, try ignorance.

Derek Bok, 25th President of Harvard University

INTRODUCTION

Building on the factors outlined in the previous chapter, the next big question to address is the cost and funding of MBAs. Whilst the cost of many MBAs may induce a sharp intake of breath, it is worth balancing this with the scholarship options presented in this chapter. Thus it may not be sufficient to simply rule out MBAs on cost basis, particularly for the over-achieving medics seeking to do MBAs in the first place!

Tuition fees in isolation range from mid £20K to over £40K per year of study (Tables 4.1 and 4.2). If support with funding is not an option, either from an employer or through a scholarship, then the potential additional out-of-pocket expense and the time over which this must be paid is important to budget for. In the main, the more expensive programmes tend to be the executive programmes based in more than one location, e.g. the Columbia University/London Business School joint highly-ranked executive programme.

Funding appears to be one of the most common explicitly 'stated' barriers to medics doing MBAs. However, marketing lessons from the MBA, discussed further in Chapter 10, advise caution about drawing such conclusions. What people *say* may be different to what people actually *do*. If, after reading this book, you decide you want to do an MBA, this chapter contains suggestions on potential sources of funding.

TIME TO BE BOLD

The best advice and ideal preparation for doing an MBA is, first, to overcome the great British reserve, and start asking and negotiating! For better or perhaps for worse, clinicians in the UK are not trained and often discouraged from talking about money. Therefore, asking for financial sponsorship for education beyond the traditional medical career path may feel awkward. However, as the discussion of financial incentives, markets and behaviour will form a large part of the MBA, the sooner you feel comfortable talking and thinking about it, the better.

In the current NHS climate, study budgets for doctors are being reduced rather than increased. Therefore, to achieve sponsorship for an MBA will require thinking 'outside of the box'. It is likely to require seeking financial support from several different pots. It is not unrealistic that gathering sufficient funding for an MBA may take several years. The sooner you can commence this process, the better. Consider offering some kind of guarantee of return to an individual or institution who agrees to sponsor you, for example, through leading on quality improvement in your department (*see* Quality Improvement Chapter 12). In addition to informal funding sources, this chapter covers formal programmes providing potential funding. The funding featured is not exhaustive but designed to challenge the assumption that the entire fee for an MBA needs to come from self-funding or an ever-dwindling NHS study budget. If employers are willing to support the MBA, then this in itself may limit the options either because of the size of the investment they are prepared to make or the caveats attached, e.g. limited days off from work or degree courses only within the UK.

Another alternative is to strategically switch employers and work for a company that is more likely to sponsor you through an MBA. This is a rather more complicated plan, as you may need to demonstrate commitment to the employer both before and after the MBA, before they will commit to funding costly postgraduate education. In addition, the process of applying for approval to do an MBA internally may be no more straightforward than some of the external sources of funding listed below. At Saïd Business School, students' employers, irrespective of whether private or public sector, fully financially sponsor only 10% of Executive MBA students. Resources and websites for further details are at the end of the chapter.

The choice, and ultimate cost, of MBA programmes is outlined in Chapter 4. One important factor is that, unlike medical schools and healthcare in general, the more you pay for an MBA the better and more highly regarded it is.

The awards discussed below are for international scholarships and UK-based sources of funding and loans.

ROTARY AMBASSADORIAL SCHOLARSHIPS

Since 1947, The Rotary Foundation has funded nearly 38 000 individuals from 100 nations to study abroad through ambassadorial scholarships. The aim of this programme is to promote international understanding and friendship between different countries. Scholarships provided include both postgraduate students and qualified professionals, such as medics.

Graham Rich, former Chief Executive of University Hospitals Bristol NHS Foundation Trust (2007–10), did an MBA at INSEAD, Fontainebleau, France 1991–92. In Graham's case, this was funded by a competitive Rotary Foundation scholarship. In exchange, he was asked to visit some French and English Rotary Clubs to speak about his experiences (Box 4.2).

FULBRIGHT MBA AWARDS

The Fulbright Commission was created in 1948, built on the legacy of the late Senator J William Fulbright: 'The simple purpose of the exchange program is to erode the culturally rooted mistrust that sets nations against one another. The exchange program is not a panacea but an avenue of hope'. Over the last 60 years, nearly 300 000 people have participated in the Fulbright Program.

Each year, one award is offered to a UK citizen specifically in support of the first year of an MBA programme, at any accredited US institution, apart from Harvard Business School considered separately below. Grants are for up to £25 000 and intended as a contribution towards the first year of tuition fees and maintenance expenses whilst in the US. This award is offered by the Fulbright Commission not just on the basis of academic excellence but also on extracurricular and community activities, ambassadorial skills, a desire to further the Fulbright Programme and a plan to give back to your home country on returning.

For MBA students at Harvard Business School, the Fulbright Commission partners with the British Friends of Harvard Business School (a registered charity) to offer 3–5 awards a year for the first year of an MBA at Harvard Business School. To be eligible, individuals must gain acceptance from Harvard before making an application. The scholarships are intended as a contribution towards the first year of tuition fees and range in value from $10 000 to $40 000.

THE THOURON AWARD

Another leading international scholarship programme is the Thouron Award, established in 1960, which now has more than 700 alumni. Graduates of British universities, including medics, can apply to become Thouron Scholars. Each year, 6–10 awards are given to British graduates who receive support for a postgraduate degree programme, such as an MBA, at the University of Pennsylvania (Wharton School of Business).

The award covers tuition fees and a monthly stipend to cover living costs, including extras such as entertainment and travel. Thouron Scholars are chosen for their academic potential and their 'ambassadorial qualities' to act as representatives of their home country. Candidates need to apply separately to the University of Pennsylvania and the Thouron Awards. Application for the Business School includes submission of GMAT scores (Chapter 6).

BANK LOANS

In the UK, NatWest currently offer loans of up to two-thirds of your annual gross pre-course salary plus course fees with a variable interest rate of 7.7%. This applies to MBAs approved by the Association of MBAs, for UK resident graduates with at least two years work experience. This can be a reasonable option if you are determined to do an MBA and are unable to find funding elsewhere.

CAREER DEVELOPMENT LOANS

Launched in 1988, Professional and Career Development Loans of up to £10 000 are available through an arrangement between the Learning and Skills Council and three high street banks (Barclays Bank, the Co-operative Bank and the Royal Bank of Scotland). This UK government sponsored scheme includes postgraduate courses, such as MBAs. There is no interest to pay on this while you are studying. However, interest rates post-qualification vary from bank to bank.

BUSINESS SCHOOL SPECIFIC FUNDING

In addition to the above funding sources, a wide range of business school specific scholarships and bursaries are available from all of the institutions and websites listed at the end of Chapter 4.

All UK and international business schools hold regular information events and open evenings where you can meet with tutors and current students. This will present you with the opportunity to ask specifically about scholarships and funding opportunities that are most appropriate for you. Scholarships often relate to increasing opportunities for applicants from specific nationalities, such as India, or backgrounds, such as engineering and technology. Specific companies often fund them. In addition, many business schools offer scholarships for women to advance their representation at senior leadership positions within industry, including those through the Forté Foundation.

An astute approach to funding is to invite a potential sponsor with you to your desired business school information event.

SUMMARY

As far as support with funding goes, if you don't ask, you don't get! Securing funding for an MBA is a test of inquisitiveness, initiative and determination. These characteristics are likely to serve you well in the commercial world.

The financial cost is not the only hurdle to beginning your MBA. The following chapter considers additional differences between medical and business schools.

FURTHER READING

Fulbright Commission. Fulbright MBA Award. www.fulbright.co.uk/fulbright-awards/for-uk-citizens/postgraduate-student-awards/mba-awards

Lifelong Learning. Career development loans. www.lifelonglearning.co.uk/cdl/

NatWest. MBA loan. www.natwest.com/personal/loans/g1/professional-training-loan/mba.ashx

Rotary International in Great Britain and Ireland (RIBI). Ambassadorial scholarships. www.ribi.org/foundation/scholarships/ambassadorial-scholarships

The Thournon Award. www.thouronaward.org/index.php?action=PublicFoundersDisplay

CHAPTER 6

The difference between choosing a business school and medical school

What's the difference between God and a surgeon?
God doesn't think he's a surgeon.

INTRODUCTION

Sometimes considered an afterthought is the MBA application requirements and application itself. The core requirements for MBAs vary along a clear theme.

Competitive barrier to entry is one of the biggest similarities between applying to business and medical schools. This criterion alone is sufficient to appeal to a certain cohort of over-achievers, characteristics not rare amongst the medical profession. In addition to the factors and cost implications outlined in Chapters 4 and 5, there are further barriers to overcome when choosing where to study an MBA that differ from the medical school experience. This chapter discusses the similarities between medical school and business school admission procedures.

MEDICAL SCHOOL

The Times Good University Guide (2010) top ten ranking institutions to study medicine has similar names to those listed in Chapter 4 as offering high ranking MBA programmes in the UK, Table 6.1.

TABLE 6.1 *The Times* Good University Guide top ten institutions to study medicine

1	Oxford		
2	Cambridge		
3	Edinburgh		
4	Aberdeen		
= 5	University College London	Imperial College	
= 7	Glasgow	Dundee	Newcastle
10	St Andrews		

Source: *The Times* online Good University Guide (2010).

In 2008, over 19 000 A-level students competed for 8000 places at UK medical schools. All applicants to study medicine at Oxford, Cambridge, Imperial and University College London (UCL) are required to sit the Biomedical Admissions Test (BMAT). Most other medical schools require candidates to sit the United Kingdom Clinical Aptitude Test (UKCAT). This tests non-cognitive abilities, similar in approach to the corporate sector. The UKCAT has been piloted since 2007. Although the results are not currently used in selection, the aim is that they will be by 2011/12. To date, the evidence suggests that the UKCAT may show a favourable bias towards men and students from a higher socioeconomic class and independent or grammar schools. It has been shown to provide a reasonable proxy for academic performance in A-levels. This is similar to the GMAT, discussed below.

BUSINESS SCHOOL

As with medicine, large numbers of international students come to the UK to study MBAs. This brings an international perspective to the MBA programme, wherever you study. However, with the benefit of age and work experience, medics looking to do MBAs in an increasingly globalised market could consider the international options shown in the global MBA rankings in Table 6.2. Some of the funding opportunities available for international study are discussed in Chapter 5.

TABLE 6.2 The *Financial Times* global top ten ranking business schools and MBAs

1	London Business School	
2	University of Pennsylvania: Wharton	
3	Harvard Business School	
4	Stanford University GSB	
5	Insead	
= 6	Columbia Business School	IE Business School
8	MIT Sloan School of Management	
= 9	University of Chicago: Booth	Hong Kong UST Business School

Source: The *Financial Times* Global Business School and MBA rankings (2010).

Choosing where to study a subject that you have only minimal insight into is difficult. Of assistance is Table 6.3. This shows the criteria that recently qualified MBA graduates would look for in choosing an MBA programme in today's climate (2009). These factors are particularly relevant as they are from people with the benefit of hindsight.

TABLE 6.3 Criteria MBA alumni would look for in a programme in today's climate

General		Curriculum		Other	
Student base	10%	Sustainability	11%	Pedagogy	20%
School ratings	26%	Ethics	9%	International dimension	8%
Accreditation	3%	Risk management	16%	Practical components	21%
Alumni association	3%	Change management	19%	Other	
		Innovation	7%	Pedagogy	20%
		Leadership	13%	International dimension	8%
		Other	33%	Practical components	21%

Source: Durham Business School and the Association of MBAs (2009).

Similar to the UKCAT, the Graduate Management Admission Test (GMAT) is a standardised assessment used by over 1900 Business Schools globally to predict future academic performance. It measures basic verbal, mathematical and analytical writing skills. It costs $250 to take at certified test centres. A high-scoring GMAT is required for entry to many MBA programmes. Box 6.1 describes one medic's experience of sitting this, prior to commencing his MBA at London Business School (LBS).

Whilst virtually all US business schools already demand the GMAT, increasingly so are European (including British) schools. Some places are content to waive the requirements if sufficient managerial experience can be demonstrated, or if the candidate has done the Graduate Record Exam (GRE) since there is considerable overlap. Increasingly, business schools are requiring certain scores on the GMAT or at least evidence of a balanced score, i.e. no paucity of skills in maths. Taking the GMAT can require considerable study as much of the exam covers topics that are long forgotten such as algebra (or even grammar rules). Whilst there are usually plenty of exam slots, it is worth forward planning since at busy periods even these slots become scarce.

BOX 6.1 Getting through GMAT

What is the chance that the next ball we draw from the bag will be blue? How long is the hypotenuse in this right-angled triangle? Where exactly should that comma go? A first glance at a GMAT paper may conjure up a rather surreal vision of what smartly suited executives spend caffeine-fuelled hours grappling with in their corporate boardrooms of the world.

Business school admission committees are faced with hundreds of applicants' essays, with tales of workplace success, of extracurricular triumph, of lofty ambition. They need some kind of objective measure to help them separate the men from the boys and the women from the girls. This is the GMAT. It tells them how well you can string a sentence (and an argument) together. It tells them whether you are as numerate as you might claim.

The GMAT has three components: analytical writing, verbal and quantitative (aka short essays, words, numbers). You take the test sitting at a computer screen. The whole thing is computer marked, including the essays, and you receive your mark straight away.

The analytical writing component involves writing two short essays. The first asks you to discuss an issue. The second asks you to analyse an argument.

(continued)

The verbal component has you doing all kinds of strange things not particularly reminiscent of any exam you have ever seen before, but most of which make sense. The three question types are 'reading comprehension', 'critical reasoning' and 'sentence correction'.

The quantitative section essentially tests how much you would embarrass yourself if you were pitched against an intelligent 16-year-old and forced to re-sit your maths GCSE today. Its content is rather quaintly described as 'arithmetic, elementary algebra and commonly known concepts of geometry'.

The test is described as 'computer-adapative'. Essentially, if you are getting questions right, the computer will ask you harder and harder questions. This allows you to prove how bright you are. If you start getting questions wrong, they will get easier again until the computer finds your level.

At the end of your three and a half hours, the kindly receptionist will hand you a computer printout that summarises your intellectual capacity (well, your GMAT-sitting capacity) in a few short numbers. You will get scores out of 800 for verbal ability, quantitative ability, and a summary score. Each of these scores has a percentile by it, telling you where you fit in the population of GMAT-test takers.

Not all business schools require the GMAT. Those that do often do not specify a particular cut-off, but consider your GMAT score alongside the rest of your application. Their websites give you some idea of previous classes' average scores.

As with medical exams, you can throw as much money at the GMAT as you like. There is no shortage of courses available. I would recommend that you at least start with the shoestring version. Google GMAT and try a few of the free practice questions. Buy any one of the numerous books of practice questions, available for about £20. Do not be intimidated by the GMAT. It is just words and numbers. You have got sufficiently far in life that the chances are that you can do these things. Depending on how good you are with words and numbers, you may not even need to do much book work. A few hours might be plenty. Good luck!

Dr Paul Rutter, LBS 2009–11

Tables 4.1 and 4.2 show that for the majority of MBA programmes, both essays and interviews are involved in the application process, as well as the GMAT.

Generally, only a small percentage of applicants are interviewed. Samples of interview questions for Harvard Business School (HBS) MBA are shown in Box 6.2, as recalled by one doctor who was successful in securing scholarships for a Masters in Public Policy (MPP) at Harvard Kennedy School as well as an MBA at HBS. Interviews for HBS MBA regularly take place in London, classically with a representative of HBS admissions committee or one professor from the business school accompanied by a human resources representative. Box 6.3 shows similar questions for MBA interviews at London Business School. The best way to prepare for these interviews is to be clear in your own mind exactly why you want to do an MBA. Next, schedule mock interviews to practise explaining your thought process to others, preferably those who will give honest objective feedback on your performance. Finessing your interview technique is a good investment of time for future job interviews. It is a skill often covered within MBA courses themselves.

BOX 6.2 Harvard Business School MBA sample questions

- What precipitated the transition between clinical practice and your current position?
- How did you cope with this transition?
- What do you think are the main challenges facing healthcare in the UK?
- How do these differ from the challenges facing the US? Do you think the UK health system is better?
- Why do you need an MBA?
- What will you bring to the HBS class?
- How do you think your perspective will add value to the class?
- What do you think you will find the most challenging part of the course?
- What do you do in your spare time/what would you like to do (out of work) if you had more time?

Source: Harvard MBA student (2010).

BOX 6.3 London Business School MBA sample questions

- Why do an MBA?
- Why come to London Business School?
- What do you see as the biggest concerns in the NHS?
- What do you want to do after your MBA?
- What do you expect to find difficult?
- What can your fellow students learn from you?
- How do you deal with stress?
- Please tell me something not on your CV, which explains why you should be accepted to London Business School.

Source: London Business School MBA student (2009).

SUMMARY

The application processes for most MBA programmes are broadly similar. The key differences are in the need for interviews and the precise nature of the questions set to probe individual interest for and aptitude at the MBA. Choosing to apply to multiple business schools in a bid to either allow chance to decide the choice or to increase the likelihood of acceptance comes at the price of multiple time-consuming forms, which often require extensive essay type responses. Thus unless there are extenuating circumstances, for example, partners applying together and thus the overriding decider about school is both being accepted, it may be more sensible to constrain the number of applications and focus on quality not quantity.

Business school, like medical school, is incredibly competitive to enter. At present, there is a more globalised market for MBAs, than for undergraduate medical school in the UK. Scoring highly in the GMAT, as well as practising interview techniques, will increase the likelihood not just of being accepted onto your desired MBA programme but also being considered for funding support through scholarship opportunities, discussed in Chapter 5.

FURTHER READING

Durham Business School and Association of MBAs (2009). *The Post Downturn MBA: an agenda for change*. London: Association of MBAs.

Financial Times. Global MBA rankings 2010. http://rankings.ft.com/businessschoolrankings/global-mba-rankings

James D, Yates J, Nicholson S (2010). Comparison of A level and UKCAT performance in students applying to UK medical and dental schools in 2006: cohort study. *BMJ*; **349**: c478.

The GMAT.® www.mba.com/mba/thegmat

The Times. The Good University Guide 2010. www.timesplus.co.uk/tto/news/?login=false&url=http://www.thetimes.co.uk/tto/education/gooduniversityguide/?subject

White C (3 March 2010). Prescribed personalities. *BMJ Careers*.

SECTION 3

Climbing the MBA mountain

What is Everest without the eyes that see it? It is the hearts of men that make it big or small.

Tensing Norgay

Robert Henrique used the analogy of climbing a mountain in his book, *Captain Smith and Company*, when describing being a member of a special unit during the Second World War. Doing an MBA can feel a little like climbing a mountain but it is important to maintain perspective on the experience. Unlike climbing Mount Everest, or fighting a war, no matter how tough doing an MBA may feel, it is extremely unlikely to kill you.

The following section is the main bulk of the book. These chapters provide both an overview and an accompaniment to what you will learn and be taught during an MBA. Chapter 7 considers the individual characteristics of the leader within organisations. The following chapters focus on understanding the mechanics of how organisations operate and the levers to improve their performance, using the example of St Anywhere, a District General Hospital (DGH) as a case study.

FURTHER READING

Henriques R (1944). *Captain Smith and Company*. Right Book Club.

The who

The only thing that gives humans their humanity is their ability to interact with fellow human beings. That is the core essence of existence, and the means of survival. We are not created to work in isolation, and anyone that tries to do so will ultimately fail. So spend your time, your energy and your money on making the team around you the best it can be. Therein lies the sustainability of success.

Dr Sneh Khemka, Medical Director, Bupa International, 2010

INTRODUCTION

Too often, clinicians feel they have ticked the leadership and management box in their medical careers by attending a two- or three-day taught course in a sheep-dip fashion. In his book *Outliers* (2008), Gladwell repeatedly refers to the '10 000-hour rule'. This is that the key to success in any field is a matter of practising a specific task for a total of around 10 000 hours. In this case, we are falling woefully short of leadership training for our clinicians.

Thousands of books about leadership are published every year. Studying leadership is a very different experience to studying medical basic sciences. The emphasis is more on discussing case studies than reviewing randomised controlled trials. However, this does not mean that there is no evidence base to learn from. By its nature, developing leadership skills is as much, if not more, about experiential rather than academic didactic learning. For many, learning how to be a more effective leader is a core motivator for doing an MBA.

Chapter 3 showed that Harvard Business School is top of the global MBA league table. Harvard Business School owns the *Harvard Business Review* (*HBR*), the staple diet of MBA students globally. *HBR* has a worldwide English circulation of over 250 000. The *HBR* is widely read by academics, executives and management consultants.

Robust research into leadership commenced with trait theories in the 1920s. This approach attempted to identify the common personality characteristics of effective leaders. The popularity of this approach diminished once extensive studies concluded only that effective leaders were either above average height or below! Recent leadership thinking focuses on contingency theory. This means leadership style that is dependent on a particular situation. However, the possibilities here are limitless, so are not much help for understanding leadership development.

This chapter identifies five seminal papers from the *HBR* that relate to leadership of people and organisations. These themes overlap with facets of the Medical Leadership Competency Framework introduced in Section 1. Some of the concepts described may seem like common sense. However, despite the obvious nature of some of the implications, the aim of this chapter is to demonstrate the origins of current leadership thinking as well as to dispel some popular myths about leadership.

FOLLOWERSHIP

To be a leader, you need followers. One of the criticisms of teaching everyone about leadership is that not everyone will be a leader. Although there is some truth in this, the model of clinicians in high performing healthcare systems, such as Kaiser Permanente, is that all clinicians are a combination of 'practitioners, partners and leaders'. While most leadership teaching tends to focus on what it means to be a leader, it is fair to say that not everyone will be or even wants to be a leader of an organisation. Kellerman (2007) writes about followers of leaders. This is particularly relevant for healthcare, where multi-disciplinary teams interact across organisational boundaries. It is not always clear who is leading, who is following and where the lines of reporting and accountability lie.

Followers are defined as 'low in the hierarchy with less power, authority and influence than their superiors. They generally go along to get along, particularly with those in higher positions'. However, followers do not always comply with those more senior to them. For example, the British Medical Association (BMA) has successfully challenged political decision-making about healthcare, for example, negotiating professional salaries and regulation.

Kellerman's categories of followers lie along a continuum of engagement from 'feeling and doing absolutely nothing' to 'being passionately committed and deeply involved'. Distinctive groups are defined as isolates, bystanders, participants, activists and diehards, shown in Figure 7.1.

At one end of the spectrum, isolates are followers who are barely aware of what is going on around them. They do not know much about their leaders nor respond to them. Paradoxically, by doing nothing, such individuals maintain the status quo and further strengthen the pre-existing leadership. Isolates are most likely to appear in large organisations, like the NHS, where senior leaders in Whitehall feel remote and irrelevant. A large proportion of isolates in an organisation may impede

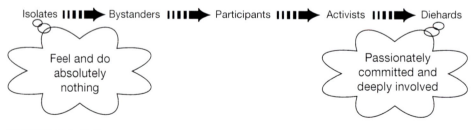

FIGURE 7.1 Followers

improvement and slow change. Engaging isolates requires individual conversations at a local level addressing individual concerns, such as job stress or job satisfaction. However, the return on such an investment may be low.

Bystanders are those that observe but do not participate. Like isolates, bystanders are passive and disengaged from leaders. Unlike isolates, bystanders are fully aware of what is going on around them; they just choose to not get involved. The bystander effect is the tendency to not intervene when a crime is being committed. As above, bystanders are commonly found in large organisations, such as the NHS. However, unlike isolates, bystanders are more likely to be incentivised to engage with the organisation to improve productivity.

Participants are those who are engaged in some way, and care enough to try and make an impact. Such individuals are incredibly valuable to organisations.

Activists are those who feel strongly about their leaders and organisations. They can be a force for or against leaders. The time and energy required means activists are frequently low in numbers. But, activists may have a substantial impact on an organisation.

Diehards display an all-consuming dedication to someone or something they consider worthy. Such individual followers are rare and can either be a strong asset to leaders or a dangerous liability. By definition, diehards are willing to risk their own health and welfare for their cause. Unlike isolates and bystanders, the opinions of diehards are crucial for leaders to be aware of.

While several of the following theories discuss the desirable attributes of good leaders, Kellerman focuses on the desired attributes of good followers. Isolates and bystanders with little or no engagement nor action, have little that is desirable to offer leaders. Good followers are those that invest their time and energy in making informed decisions about who their leaders are and what they stand for. Bad followers are those that either do nothing to contribute or actively oppose a leader that stands for good.

The key messages from Kellerman are that followers are on a spectrum of engagement. They hold power and influence in organisations, as much as leaders do. The technological advances, described in Chapter 10, mean that online networks are now increasingly able to aggregate followers and enhance their influential power.

WHY SHOULD ANYONE BE LED BY YOU?

Vision, authority and strategic direction are commonly associated with successful leadership. In their paper, Goffee and Jones (2000) identify four further qualities essential to leadership. These are:
➤ Reveal your weaknesses.
➤ Rely heavily on intuition to know how and when to act.
➤ Manage people with tough empathy.
➤ Demonstrate uniqueness by revealing differences.

Following more than 25 years of research into leaders who inspired people by capturing their hearts and minds, Goffee and Jones found that leaders with all of the above qualities were truly inspirational. A combination of all of the above is critical, mixing and matching qualities using the right style for the right moment. This is effective leadership: knowing what to use and when.

Sharing selective weaknesses as a leader makes people relate to you and creates a sense of trust. However, it must be done carefully so that a major flaw is not revealed that could jeopardise your role. Another strategy, familiar in job interviews, is to reveal a weakness that is in some ways a strength, such as being a workaholic. One of the challenges with attempting to follow Goffee and Jones' model is to do so in a way that is genuine. If a leader attempts to expose vulnerability in a disingenuous manner, this will only serve to alienate followers, as observed in politicians.

Being able to sense the mood of people in the room is an incredibly powerful leadership skill. This sense of empathy is explored further in Goleman's theories below. Being able to read silences and pick up on non-verbal cues, without being over-sensitive, guides an effective leader about when to act.

Goffee and Jones describe tough empathy as giving people what they need, rather than what they want. This approach pushes individuals to be the best they can be. Although sounding rather military in approach, tough empathy tends to be used by people who are passionate and really care about something. When people care passionately about something, others are more likely to follow.

The final facet, described by Goffee and Jones, is that of daring to be different and capitalising on such differences. Whether the difference is in style of dress, imagination or expertise, most people hesitate to shout about what sets them apart. Over time, individual leaders recognise what it is about themselves that sets them apart. The most effective leaders learn how to use their uniqueness to their advantage to inspire others to perform better. However, this does not always result in them winning a popularity contest.

Unfortunately the observations described by Goffee and Jones cannot be copied mechanically like a recipe for great leadership. Herein lies the challenge of teaching leadership. The best advice given for leaders is to be themselves – with more skill. By this, the authors mean sensitively varying what is required from context to context. And to do this compatibly with what is already naturally part of an individual's personality, as a personal style that works for you.

WHAT MAKES A LEADER?

If leadership is more of an art than a science, Goleman (1998) believes that emotional intelligence is the key to making a great leader. Table 7.1 explains what is meant by the five core components of emotional intelligence. Analysing senior managers in 188 companies, Goleman assessed three categories of capabilities: technical skills such as accounting; cognitive abilities such as analytical reasoning; and emotional intelligence, which includes working with others to lead change. For jobs at all levels, Goleman found emotional intelligence to be twice as important as the other categories. He also found that emotional intelligence played an increasingly important role at the highest levels of the company.

TABLE 7.1 Emotional intelligence

	Definition	Hallmarks
Self-awareness	Able to recognise and understand own moods, emotions and drives as well as their effect on others.	Self-confidence. Realistic self-assessment. Self-deprecating sense of humour.
Self-regulation	Able to control mood and think before acting.	Trustworthy and integrity. Comfortable with ambiguity. Open to change.
Motivation	Passionate about working beyond money or status. Pursues goals with energy and persistence.	Strong drive to achieve. Optimism, even when failure threatens. Committed to the organisation.
Empathy	Understands the emotional make up of others and skilled in treating people according to their emotional reactions.	Expertise in nurturing and retaining talent. Cross-cultural sensitivity. Excellent service to clients.
Social skill	Proficient at managing relationships and building networks. Able to find common ground and build rapport.	Effective at leading change. Persuasive. Expertise in building and leading teams.

Source: Goleman D. (1998) What makes a leader? *Harvard Business Review.*

Whilst the above characteristics may seem common sense, what is less straightforward is the debate about to what extent emotional intelligence can be learnt. Although there is an inherited component to emotional intelligence, psychological research suggests that nurture – through research and practise – plays a role.

Emotional intelligence increases with age, in line with maturity. Contrary to popular belief, enhancing emotional intelligence cannot occur by attending a one-day seminar or through self-help books. Unfortunately, there is no such thing as a fast-track emotional intelligence booster. The most effective approach to developing emotional intelligence requires motivation, extended practise and feedback. As Ralph Waldo Emerson wrote, 'Nothing great was ever achieved without enthusiasm'. The evidence suggests an individualised approach to training is recommended to break old habits and establish new ones, in keeping with Gladwell's 10 000-hour rule mentioned previously.

NARCISSISTIC LEADERS

To date, healthcare leaders lag behind other sectors in maximising their status and influence as celebrities. Healthcare leaders are less likely than others to hire publicists and appear on the covers of magazines. Looking forward, it seems likely that healthcare leaders will increasingly embrace this publicly visionary and charismatic form of leadership to deliver important healthcare messages. This may be described as narcissistic behaviour, arising from Sigmund Freud's observation that 'people of this type impress others as being "personalities" . . . They are especially suited to act as a support for others, to take on the role of leaders, and to give a fresh stimulus to cultural development or damage the established state of affairs'.

Maccoby considers the positive and negative consequences of narcissistic leadership. Leaders, known as 'productive narcissists', are able to see the bigger picture and find meaning in changing the world and establishing their legacy. Being able to see the bigger picture allows a compelling vision to be created. To quote George Bernard Shaw: 'Some people see things as they are and ask why; narcissists see things that never were and ask why not'. Productive narcissists are both risk takers and charmers. The downfalls are that they may also be unrealistic and prone to paranoia. Their ability to be skilled orators further enhances their ability to attract followers.

Narcissists are often sensitive to criticism and, for this reason, will tend to keep their own and others' emotions at arm's length. Another characteristic flaw of narcissists is their reluctance to listen. Contrary to Goleman's observations about the importance of emotional intelligence, narcissistic leaders tend to lack empathy. Narcissistic leaders are inspirational because of their passion and conviction, rather than their all too often absent touchy-feely nature. They can be exploitative and competitive, with a tendency to instruct rather than coach or mentor subordinates.

There is limited evidence for how to extract the benefits of narcissistic leadership whilst avoiding the pitfalls. Despite the risks, it may be that the ability of narcissistic leaders to create the future, rather than anticipate it, is the disruptive innovation required for healthcare today.

HOW LEADERS CREATE AND USE NETWORKS

In 2007, the *New England Journal of Medicine* published a seminal paper examining the causation and management of obesity. Controversially, Christakis and Fowler demonstrated that obesity is contagious through networks. These findings have been robustly reproduced in other populations.

A 'network' is a set of nodes – where connections are made either through individuals or organisational units – and linkages between them. Networks operate on the basis of formal and informal relationships. Through these connections and relationships, networks are made up of clusters of nodes geared towards a particular goal.

In the US, medical social networks are beginning to have more influence over clinical practice than traditional medical professional organisations. Networks, and the ability to network, matter not just for career enhancement but ultimately for improving patient care. Cross and Parker (2004) found that high performers within organisations have larger, more diversified networks than average performers. Contrary to how doctors are trained, networking is as important in healthcare as in any other sector. The advantages of being an effective networker include: being more likely to have your ideas taken up, career mobility, further contacts and more discretionary time to yourself and desired projects or research.

> The networks we rely on in a stable job are rarely the ones that lead us to something new and different. It is important to conduct our 'role rehearsals' for our

new working identity outside our usual circles because the old audience tend to narrowly typecast us.

(Herminia Ibarra, Professor of Organisational Behaviour at Insead, 2003)

Ibarra and Hunter (2007) followed 30 managers through a leadership transition, defined as an inflection point in their careers that challenged them to think about both themselves and their roles. MBAs classically induce inflection points and leadership transitions. For many aspiring leaders, clinical or not, networking can feel an uncomfortable prospect. Hence inclusion here, as an MBA both exposes students to and dispels fear from the experience of online and offline networking.

Ibarra and Hunter discuss three forms of networking: operational, personal and strategic. These three types are not mutually exclusive. Operational networking serves to assist management skills in your current role. Operational networks include all those within your current team. They also include suppliers, distributors and customers. In healthcare, operational networks include the patient as well as traversing the boundaries of health and social care, primary and secondary care. Operational networks often serve to meet the task at hand rather than thinking more strategically about what 'should' be done.

Personal networking takes place through professional associations, alumni groups and clubs. In healthcare, this may include attending lectures and/or participating with think tank meetings, such as The King's Fund and the Nuffield Trust, London. This allows new perspectives to be gained, which may aid career advancement into horizons beyond the immediate organisation. In addition to personal development, personal networking lays the foundation for strategic networking.

Strategic networking is about sourcing information, support and resources from one sector of a network, to achieve results in another. Strategic networkers may use indirect influence, convincing one person in their network to persuade someone else, not in their network, to take action. Networking takes time and, to be most effective, an operational network needs to evolve into a strategic one. One of the best ways to broaden networks is with the support of a role model or mentor.

Networking by its nature involves 'work'. Those who do it well seek every opportunity to engage with their networks whether they actually 'need' to or not. This constitutes a 'leadership network'. For such a network to thrive, participants should enjoy and want to be part of it. In the corporate sector, networking is a necessary component of leadership roles. Future healthcare leaders will be unable to avoid networking; no matter how uncomfortable or unnatural it may initially feel.

ONLINE NETWORKS

The final section of this chapter provides a brief overview of online networks. Online networks tend to traverse or rather bulldoze over personal and professional boundaries. Currently the king of all online networks is Facebook, founded in 2004 by Mark Zuckerberg. Facebook is a global networking site with over 400 million users. Between June 2008 and June 2009, Facebook's unique audience grew by a staggering 198%! However, the quality of actual networking per se on Facebook can be rather poor.

Another popular site, launched prior to Facebook in 2003, is LinkedIn.com. LinkedIn has over 65 milllion members in more than 200 countries. LinkedIn is specifically designed to facilitate professional networking and has a more self-promotional approach. It is often used in recruitment and may be useful when researching individual's backgrounds. LinkedIn, like Facebook, can be accessed from mobile phones. Both sites offer special interest groups where you can 'chat' with others.

Twitter was created in 2006. It is a social microblogging site. Individuals produce short 140-character updates called tweets. As twitter.com operates in real time, it can be used to monitor trends. Of note, the *New Scientist* (2008) reported that sites such as twitter were more effective at information dissemination than traditional news channels.

SUMMARY

The themes and articles discussed in this chapter may raise more questions than they answer. One of the main messages is that the development of leadership and management skills is a journey, rather than a box to be ticked once dipped into.

To accompany the leadership journey, this chapter has emphasised the value of understanding followership. In addition to providing an overview of the dangers of narcissistic leadership, and the benefits of emotional intelligence, it is clear that leadership is not a 'lone ranger' activity. To provide the best possible care for patients, it is not only desirable but essential that clinical leaders, and aspiring clinical leaders, are active members of and contributors to strategic networks, both on and offline.

FURTHER READING

Christakis NA, Fowler JH (2007). The spread of obesity in a large social network over 32 years. *New England Journal of Medicine*; **357**: 377–9.

Christakis NA, Fowler JH (2010). *Connected: the amazing power of social networks and how they shape our lives*. New York: HarperPress.

Cohn JM, Khuruna R, Reeves L (2005). Growing talent as if your business depended on it [extract]. *Harvard Business Review*; 63–70.

Cross R, Parker A (2004). *The Hidden Power of Social Networks: how work really gets done in organisations*. Boston: Harvard Business School Publications.

Gladwell M (2008). *Outliers: the story of success*. New York: Penguin.

Goffee R, Jones G (2000). Why should anyone be led by you? *Harvard Business Review*; 63–70.

Goleman D (1998). What makes a leader? *Harvard Business Review*; 93–102.

Ibarra H, Hunter M (2007). How leaders create and use networks. *Harvard Business Review*; 40–7.

Kellerman B (2007). What every leader needs to know about followers. *Harvard Business Review*; 84–91.

Maccoby M (2000). Narcissistic leaders: the incredible pros and cons. *Harvard Business Review*; 69–77.

CHAPTER 8

Understanding the market of healthcare

The only way that has ever been discovered to have a lot of people co-operate together voluntarily is through the free market. And that's why it's so essential to preserving individual freedom.

Milton Friedman

INTRODUCTION

When the NHS was founded in 1948, the principles that it was publically funded and free for all at the point of delivery were clear. The ethos of the NHS was to provide equitable healthcare to all who needed it. The system developed drew on European and American examples of public or 'not-for-profit' healthcare systems. The last 60 odd years have seen these principles held dear, despite rising costs and increasing demand. Over the last six decades, successive governments have tinkered with both how the NHS receives monies (although not how it is funded), and by whom care is delivered. Both have occurred in part to save resources and in part to drive up quality, perhaps complicated by the need to do so within political ideologies.

The current state of the NHS is perhaps best described as a public system with market mechanisms at play. These market mechanisms were not passive evolution but rather were created through active encouragement. Some argue they have gone too far. Others argue that they have not gone far enough. The marketisation of the NHS occurred because of a belief shared by the two major political parties that markets drive efficiency and quality. A true market for healthcare would need to accept consequences such as market failures. This might mean hospitals becoming bankrupt or that inequalities might increase. Because of these risks, the introduction of market principles has occurred in such a way as to perpetuate strong public control. Thus, the perception by some that the evolution has been too slow and by others that it has gone too far.

This chapter is an overview of how the market applies to healthcare in the UK at present. The aim of this chapter is to allow those focused on provision of care to better understand how to influence those around them to ensure that the services they support flourish. In part this comes from understanding the landscape, but also from examining some of the levers of change. Ultimately, success in translating the big picture to be relevant to the individual service relies on using the tools of the organisation for making the case for change through writing a business plan. The final section of this chapter is an examination of how to structure a business case.

IS THE NHS A MARKET OR NOT?

The classic definition of a market is simple: 'a place where goods or services or information may be exchanged'. Unlike Scotland, where there has been limited implementation of market reforms. Perhaps the most important change of the last 20 years has been the increasing division within England of healthcare providers from commissioners. This creates a fundamental of the market: sellers and buyers. However, the purchasers of care are not those who are directly using the care; instead purchasing is done on behalf of local populations by organisations, with special skills and responsibilities. The problem with this set up is that it creates an agency problem, i.e. are the interests of those purchasing care aligned with the needs and demands of those who will actually receive care?

Providers are those who deliver care either in acute or primary care settings (and indeed increasingly with integrated care options across the acute and primary care division). This embraces both hospitals and smaller organisations such as community nurses through ambulance trusts. Commissioners are those that buy the care. Until recently in England, this has been Primary Care Trusts (PCT). Looking ahead, this function will be overseen by groups of GPs. To date, there is almost complete disassociation between purchasers and providers, except that some PCTs have yet to finally divest their provider arm. Perversely, and perhaps increasingly importantly, GPs may act as both providers and commissioners through practice-based commissioning.

Purchasers and providers are not enough to create a market place unless there is a mechanism to enable funding to flow in the marketplace. For example, a cattle market without money flowing between the buyers and sellers would not work. Thus a construct called 'Payment by Results' was instituted to accompany patient choice. In the main, when a patient goes to a hospital, the PCT receives a bill after the patient has been treated (based on the coding from the admission, as entered into HES – the Information Technology system). Then the PCT would reimburse the hospital (albeit at an aggregated level). One of the many challenges of the market in healthcare surrounds the price.

HOW DO YOU COST THE PROVISION OF CARE, AND HOW TO CHARGE FOR IT?

The introduction of 'Payment by Results' (PBR) means that the cost of any procedure is based on the average cost of provision. However, few providers are confident of their costs. Equally, many argue that charging on this basis disincentivises good purchasing for a variety of reasons. In most true markets, the price is set at the intersection of the point that the purchasers are willing to pay and the providers can afford to sell. PBR does not allow the market to acclimatise the price; rather it is imposed. The price may encompass the wrong thing. For example, at present the price is based on isolated episodes of care, or procedures, not on bundles of care or years of care provision. Clearly prices that include more risk borne by the provider have the potential to reduce cost. One such mechanism is seen in use by Geisinger Health in Pennsylvania. Here, the hospital charges a fixed rate for surgeries, e.g. coronary angioplasty. If the patient has a complication, the hospital bears the cost rather than the insurer being asked to pay again for another admission, as would happen in the UK. Such a costing schedule has meant that Geisinger has been incentivised to improve the quality of care it provides, and thereby reducing such complications. This is achieved through strict enactment of American College of Cardiology Guidelines and also that the price for the surgery was calculated based on clear understanding of the cost structure. This is something that few hospitals in the UK can so far achieve.

A third important factor in creating markets in health is competition. Competition is the mechanism by which the market generates the drive to efficiency and quality. Purchasers choose the better value or higher quality provision thus, in theory, reducing flow to costly or ineffective services. Competition has thus seen the NHS shift from a monopoly towards a more open market place, although it would be hard at present to call it an oligopoly, let alone a market. The potential for competition is created at the provider level. Although PCTs may buy care either through the NHS, third sector or private sector, the amount that can be paid for such care is often fixed. As explained earlier in the chapter, procedures or clinician interactions are priced via PBR. This is a national system that creates a tariff for episodes of care. Conditions or procedures not yet covered by the tariff are funded by local agreements between PCT and provider. The tariff may vary between geographic locations but the money still follows the patient.

To date, there has been no real competition at the purchaser level. Money flows from Strategic Health Authorities (SHA) to PCTs, who use the money to purchase care on behalf of their population. Even practice-based commissioning uses soft budgeting. This means that they spend allocated amounts without suffering the consequence of overspend, as the PCT is still ultimately accountable for the money. In other countries, e.g. the USA and perhaps more useful for comparison purposes Holland or Germany, commissioning is also a market through the creation of a number of bodies able to purchase care on behalf of their populations. This means that the public can choose who they will use as their agent to argue and negotiate the best value and quality care for them. As with car insurance, the idea is that those buying insurance are able to shop around and find the product that works best for them. Competition thus drives the insurers to create better deals for customers to attract custom. To facilitate this in the UK would require a fundamental shift, since at present money does not follow individuals when it comes to commissioning. Instead, the equivalent of insurers – the commissioners or PCTs – are funded based on a population-based risk adjustment using the resource allocation formula. The Department of Health (DH) gives PCTs across the country a set amount every year to buy care for their local population based on certain factors, e.g. age of people in their population, sex, etc. To move to a system where there was competition would require the government to give the money to buy care to the patient, and then they would choose their insurer. This is highly complex, not least because so doing would require the government to be able to work out how much the basic sum given to patients should be and how much extra they should pay for risky patients, i.e. the elderly or already sick; otherwise the insurers would not want sick patients. This is possible, as Holland and Germany have shown. Interestingly, this system seems to lead to high levels of satisfaction amongst users – perhaps because they feel more in control. To a certain extent, this is occurring in a limited trial in the UK for patients with long-term conditions who have been given personal health budgets, which they can use to buy services directly. The evidence that patients holding their own healthcare budgets will make decisions that will lead to the best outcomes is mixed, although the use of decision-making aids has been shown to enhance patient outcomes. The difference in the UK is that the middlemen (the insurers), who can secure better deals because they negotiate on behalf of many and thus benefit from economies of scale and scope, are not involved.

Another key market element that is still underdeveloped in the UK is information exchange. In most markets, information is key. Imagine buying a car: to get the best deal requires the purchaser to consider their preferred features and then to shop around different brands and/or companies to find the best deal for them. Until very recently, patients were unable to do this. Now there are information sources such as the NHS Choices website.

Thus increasingly the market consists of those buying services and those providing them. The presence of such a market is hoped to act as a lever for improving quality and reducing cost. The question that vexes politicians, health economists, policy makers and health service researchers, not to mention the public, patients and clinicians, is: is it true that the market achieves this? Is it true that choice and allowing resources to follow the patient improve care?

The British Medical Association (BMA) clearly feels that the marketisation of the NHS has gone too far and is compromising clinical care. Advocates of the market reform argue that recent relaxations of monopolistic powers have led to less inequality, and that competition has improved outcomes. Perhaps the fairest assessment is that it is too soon to answer this question within the unique UK context, since the structural reforms to enable this set up are still relatively new, and comparison to other countries means that the specific circumstances of the UK are not comparable (even with complicated statistical adjustments). Perhaps instead, the effect of becoming a system with market mechanisms at play is that the language of health has shifted. Today, people talk of competition, of demand and supply, of costs (and even activity-based costing – where costs are explored through basic units, e.g. cost of knee replacement), to name but a few. *See* Box 8.1 for a breakdown of some key economic phrases.

BOX 8.1 Key economics definitions

AVERAGE COST is the total cost divided by the total output (TC/Q), for example, the total cost of care for all hip replacements carried out divided by the total number of patients treated. Average costs tend to fall as output increases, called ECONOMIES OF SCALE. However, beyond a certain point, the average cost starts to rise with output. This is called DISECONOMIES OF SCALE or decreasing returns and shows that large size is not always an advantage.

BARRIERS TO ENTRY are obstacles that may make it difficult to enter a specific market.

'A barrier to entry is anything that prevents entry when entry is socially beneficial' (Fisher, FM. (1979). *Diagnosing Monopoly.*)

CAPACITY refers to the point of production, or number of patients treated, at which a company or organisation's costs begin to rise because of a fixed factor such as number of treatment rooms or healthcare staff.

DEMAND is the quantity buyers wish to buy at each price, for example, the amount of care required for a given population with diabetes that the PCT will pay the hospital for. In a true market, low prices create excess demand.

ECONOMIES OF SCOPE are similar to economies of scale, but instead of looking at supply-side changes, such as varying the output, economies of scope refer to efficiencies with demand-side changes. This includes GPs offering a broader range of services, such as minor procedures, at a local level within clinics.

FIXED COST are costs whose size is independent of the level of activity, for example, the salary of the CEO of a hospital trust. For public services, it is possible for fixed costs to be sunk (as below), unless the monopoly is regulated.

MARGINAL COST is the cost of producing one additional unit, or treating one additional patient. This refers to the incremental cost per individual and is different to the average cost. If the marginal cost is below the average cost, the average cost falls as output rises. Once marginal cost is above the average cost, it follows that average cost rises as output rises.

MONOPOLY is a market structure in which a single seller of a product with no close substitutes serves the entire market. The absence of choice and competition means that the price ends up being higher than it would be with choice. As in the NHS, this situation may be inefficient and means there is a lack of incentives to innovate.

PRICE DISCRIMINATION is selling at different prices to different customers, as in peak and off-peak train fares. An example from healthcare is out-of-hours GP services who may sell their contracts at different rates to different GP surgeries or PCTs. In addition, patients admitted to NHS wards are able to pay an additional charge to have their own private room, replicating the model of business class versus economy class.

PRICE ELASTICITY is a measure for the responsiveness, or elasticity, of the quantity demanded of a service or product to a change in its price. For example, demand is said to be inelastic if any changes in the price of a service have a relatively small impact on the amount of the service required. Demand is said to be elastic if changes in price lead to a large effect in the amount of service demanded. Commissioning seeks to increase the elasticity of healthcare costs.

SUNK COST are costs that cannot be recovered by reversing or changing decisions. Economic decisions should be forward thinking: 'Let bygones be bygones'.

SUPPLY is the quantity producers wish to sell at each price, for example, the amount of outpatients appointments a clinic can provide to treat cataracts. In a true market, high prices lead to excess supply.

TOTAL COST includes both fixed and variable costs (TC).

VARIABLE COST: Costs whose size varies with activity level, for example, treating more patients in Accident and Emergency departments is likely to cost the hospital more money.

Whilst theory is important, and an MBA stretches knowledge of theory, fundamental to understanding is the ability to link the concepts described in Box 8.1 to the day-to-day reality. This chapter has touched on the concept of the market and how this has affected healthcare provision in the UK. The next section looks at a specific example of a service and focuses on how these forces shape the way the service is acting, in particular focusing on the levers of the market.

THE SERVICE

St Anywhere is a moderate size District General Hospital (DGH). It is served by two PCTs, both of which are struggling financially. The hospital sits on the outskirts of a large town, and has old building stock with a Private Finance Initiative (PFI) build about to come online. The Ophthalmology service faces serious competition from two local sources: one, an out branch of the best locally renowned eye hospital and two, a strong DGH nearby. The Ophthalmology service has been through various iterations over the last 10 years: partnerships with other local DGHs, 'tie ins' with the leading local eye centre and a period where it looked like the service might be closed completely.

Currently the clinics are bursting with patients – both internal referrals, for example, from the diabetic screening service and external referrals. The big question is whether to expand the service or not and if extra services should be offered.

The lead clinician feels there is a case for expansion, i.e. increasing the number of medical and nursing (alongside technical and administrative) staff based on HES data. For the hospital, this means considerable investment in people on a long-term basis since jobs are rarely time-limited in the NHS. To enable a functional service there will need to be a capital investment in equipment and data housing.

Further improvements in productivity and efficiency can be achieved to reduce the capital investment to the minimum, using metrics like new to follow-up ratio, Did Not Attend (DNA) rates, average appointment times, clinic capacity and templates. The lead clinician working with the Quality Improvement (QI) team plans to focus on these improvements and balance the gains by measuring satisfaction pre-implementation with a plan to re-survey post-implementation of both staff and patients.

The lead clinician at St Anywhere knows that if he can generate more revenue and improve measurable quality, this will act as a virtuous circle. This is because St Anywhere is in the vanguard of hospitals that have adopted service-line management and service-line reporting. In essence, this means that the ophthalmology service is acting as an autonomous business unit. The lead clinician in association with a general manager is accountable and responsible for the unit budget. Every year they negotiate with the hospital how much of their surplus they must handover to the hospital (in addition to monies to cover overheads) and what their goals should be. If they are able to meet their goals (both financial and other), and provide their contribution margin, a proportion of the surplus is theirs to reinvest in their service. Success means that the service grows and benefits. Where this has been implemented in England, it has increased clinician engagement in management and helped to ensure that productivity, efficiency and quality improvement go hand in hand.

This short snapshot mirrors what happens regularly throughout England. It exemplifies a number of issues. First, that the normal lever of increasing throughput is not applicable in the NHS because there are finite resources. Second, that unlike in other markets, competition cannot occur solely on price, since the main price is fixed. Instead, competition has to occur on cost. This is being driven actively by the Department of Health gently altering the tariff. Ophthalmology is in the vanguard of this push, since the pathways of care are well worked out. In the 2010–11 tariff, instead of cataract surgery being paid for, in addition to every outpatient appointment there is now a bundled price, meaning that hospitals are being encouraged and incentivised to improve their efficiency. This means that to continue to provide the pathway without losing money, the pathway needs to be altered. Under the set up most hospitals currently employ, this would not occur; therefore services need to redesign along the lines laid out earlier, thereby achieving a lower cost base and increased quality of care.

The above example also highlights the role of information. The referral practice is likely to change, based not on whim but on information. If St Anywhere can either provide information showing its competitive advantages or simply be the place to go to for general information, it is likely to attract more business. Either way, information provision is likely to require provision of data and this in turn may well drive up quality. Showing benchmarked data to clinicians has been demonstrated to drive their competitive spirit. A further important lever that this scenario identifies is the agency factor. In this scenario, the patient is being supported to make decisions by PCT choices and GP practice. Assuring alignment for all of this with the patients' interest is tricky. Increasingly, patient panels are supporting PCT choices. In addition, 'choose and book' and improved patient- and public-orientated information websites allow more input from the patient. To date, there have been limited attempts to directly market services to patients, although other countries do allow this. To do this would bring benefits as well as disadvantages.

The final section of this chapter looks at how the lead clinician in the St Anywhere example can make his case to the Executive Board to allow the expansion he believes is crucial to the viability and quality of his service.

For clinicians, the currency of persuasion is evidence-based medicine. The last 30 years have seen an acceptance of the argumentative power of odds ratios and p values. Clinicians have become adept at altering practice on the basis of new studies or meta-analysis, rightly relying on the skills of the few who have become adept at such interpretation, e.g. Cochrane reviews. Managers too have a language of persuasion: the business case. Whilst this may be frustrating to clinicians, and the language unintelligible in many ways, the key to success is translating between these worlds. Perhaps there is a bigger argument to be had over where responsibility lies for this; in the renowned Mayo Clinic, for example, responsibility would lie with administrators who facilitate clinical decision-making. In England, the responsibility is perhaps more evenly spread; in some institutions it is perhaps placed more on the clinician.

Business cases take many forms, in part dependent on the exact scenario in question, to which the case is being pitched, and the form, i.e. in person or on paper. Most institutions have formulaic templates that are often very frustrating and deeply repetitive. In fact, some make communicating key messages harder rather than easier, not least because of the length of the eventual plan (which puts off all but the most lionhearted).

However, the essence of the case is fairly fixed. The case is really a bird's eye view of the landscape in which the change is happening – looking at the economic reality, alongside a detailed explanation of why the change is needed and what the change will look like both qualitatively and quantitatively.

The key areas are: an executive summary (akin to the abstract of a paper), the change that is to occur, who will be overseeing the change, the current market and competition, how the change will be marketed, how the change will be operationalised, the timescale, finances and then the opportunities and risks. A variation on the above would be that there were a number of options and these would each need to be considered in turn. Detail about the process of change management itself is discussed in Chapter 11.

Using the St Anywhere example as a case study, the nuances can be explored further. Below is a shortened version of the sort of case that an executive team would hope to see to allow them to decide whether to invest.

St Elsewhere Business Case example

Executive summary

St Anywhere Ophthalmology seeks to maintain and grow their service. To date, the service has provided the highest contribution margin of any service (over 50% of revenue). Recent modelling shows that at present, demand is exceeding capacity in particular with outpatient follow-up appointments. Examining the market, it is clear that it is a growing market due to demographic change (ageing population) and that St Anywhere is currently losing market share to its competitors. Thus there is potential to increase throughput without increasing PCT spend, rather by repatriating services to St Anywhere from competitors. The ophthalmology service believes that this fits both with national, local and hospital policy since it will allow patients high quality care closer to home. Furthermore, the service believes that the surplus generated can be increased through efficiencies of scope and scale alongside productivity gains from reform of pathways.

This business case provides information concerning three potential options. First, do nothing: this means that further market share will be lost. Additionally the lack of capital investment in equipment means that patients will suffer from sub-standard care and the potential overstretch of staff increases the risk of error and patient harm. The second option is phased expansion, first an increase to four consultants from the current three with a concurrent increase in non-consultant staffing, nursing and administrative support. The cost of this increase (Z) would be balanced by the projected increase in revenue generated since this increase in capacity would allow X increase in patients to be seen, generating Y income assuming the same case mix. The second phase of this option would, after 18 months to two years, be to add a further consultant and ancillary team. This team would specifically focus on certain core pathways of work, rather than general work, since it is clear that the demography and ethnicity of the area demands it, plus the lack of a local service. National Institute for Clinical Excellence (NICE) and PCT guidance means that this too has clear revenue-generating potential alongside improving care for patients who currently must seek this service at great geographic distance from home. The third option is to do the two phases of option 2 at once. Both option 2 and 3 require capital investment to support the staff expansion, funding for picture storage and further investment in equipment.

The change

The ophthalmology service is proposing expansion in staff to allow market share capture. Current modelling shows that present demand is already exceeding supply (capacity). Expansion will thus allow the ability to meet current demand and indeed to recapture market share from local competitors both in general ophthalmology and, ideally, specific areas not well served at present, e.g. retinal work. It is clear that increasing staff cannot be the sole mechanism by which the service generates revenue. National policy (and indeed pricing via the tariff) and focus on the patient needs mean that concurrently there should be gains in productivity and efficiency, e.g. decreasing the new to follow-up ratio, DNA rates and altering care pathways to reduce the need for hospital visits. Furthermore, a high proportion of costs arise from utilisation of hospital-based facilities investment in people, e.g. community optometrist and the use of new venues such as polyclinics are further ways to reduce expenses and improve the quality of care. The combination of these efforts will lead to a larger, more efficient, more stimulating environment to work in that is able to best provide for the needs of the local community.

Oversight

The team developing and instituting the proposal are a multi-professional team of ophthalmologists, opticians, orthoptists, nurses and indeed patients (via a patient forum). This multi-professional team is ideally placed to ensure that the needs of the local population are met and that the most up-to-date practice is incorporated. Equally, having a team set up means that productivity gains arising from altered work patterns are more feasible.

The current market and competition

An ageing population with a highly diverse ethnic mix means that the prevalence and indeed incidence of eye disease in the population that St Anywhere serves is likely to increase. For example, glaucoma rates are expected to increase by 20% over 10 years. Thus the market is growing. However, demand is likely to be managed, e.g. by increasing the thresholds for operations, since PCTs are unlikely to increase spend dramatically due to the global economic picture and the micro level situation. For the ophthalmology service at St Anywhere to remain viable, i.e. able to provide patients with high quality care in a cost effective manner, constant improvement is required.

Ophthalmology has seen recent technological advances that translate to the need for new equipment and new data storage, e.g. for retinal photographs. Maintaining such a service requires economies of scale and scope and thus growth. Growth, as shown, will not come from increased flow, at least in the short-term, unless this is market share capture. The current competitors have comparative advantages over St Anywhere:

the out branch of the local eye hospital has a great reputation. The adjacent DGH has had considerable recent investment and thus appears a highly marketable option. Furthermore, because of this investment they are able to offer more timely appointments, thus benefiting through 'choose and book'. It is likely that at least one of the competitors will rise to meet the challenge and the adjacent PCT may struggle to focus on this since they are at present undergoing a re-organisation and merger. Thus the key to success will be marketing the message around St Anywhere.

St Anywhere will be seeking to increase throughput by repatriating patient care, i.e. re-capturing lost market share in general ophthalmology, and to meet the needs of an underserved segment of the population, those with retinal disease. The major barrier to entry in this part of the market is the cost of staff, skills and equipment.

This marketing section would include clear projections for growth in terms of patients, converted to approximations of revenue and market share recapture, ideally visually.

How will the change be marketed?

To regain market share requires more than just staff and equipment. It requires clear communication to the local population (through GPs and PCTs) that the service is refreshed and uniquely placed to meet the specific needs of the population. A particular comparative advantage of St Anywhere is that it is a DGH, i.e. patients can be seen on site for multiple diseases concurrently, whereas visiting the local out branch of the eye hospital does not allow this. The new PFI building provides a wonderful opportunity to invite GPs and the public to see the new facilities. If this is coupled with renewed efforts to build relationships, this could be a powerful marketing campaign. Indeed, it may be decided that it is advantageous to focus the target market into those GPs who are currently referring beyond St Anywhere.

How will the change be operationalised?

This operational section would contain details of new pathway designs showing efficiency savings and increases in productivity. This would sit alongside conceptualisation of the anticipated changes to the location of care delivery. Thus it might be that the new average consultant week, using polyclinics, might exemplify this. This section would also detail the equipment required. Furthermore, this section would provide supplementary support from patients and patients groups. Equally, this section would be where the evidence from the demand and capacity analysis might sit, including sensitivity analysis. This is a technique akin to scenario modelling (where different visions for the future are generated to help planning) where difference values are inputted into models to estimate the maximum and minimum gain or loss. In this case, the models may look at alternative staff arrangements including the expansion of non-consultant staff.

Timescale

A detailed timescale, perhaps using a GANT chart would be included. Fundamental to this is building in milestones, which are key deliverables against which performance can be judged. It makes sense to ensure that the early deliverables are relatively easy to achieve, since it is demoralising to all (and unhelpful) particularly in a phased set up if early milestones are missed.

Finances

This finance section is best explored using comparative tables. In particular, it is imperative to clearly outline the expected costs, the revenues (and the assumptions behind these calculations) as well as the break-even points. Clearly these numbers are not likely to be perfect but they show that the financial background is understood and best use of available numbers are made.

TABLE 8.1 Finance projections example

	Patients seen broken into outpatient (new and follow up/elective surgeries)	Income – using tariff	Expenditure (broken into pay and non-pay e.g. drugs/ equipment/overheads	Surplus + or –
Year 1				
Year 2				
Etc.				

Opportunities and risk

One mechanism to assess opportunities and risk is to perform a SWOT analysis. This framework allows examination of the strengths, weaknesses, opportunities and threats. This approach is also used in Chapter 10.

TABLE 8.2 SWOT analysis

Strengths	Creates a robust flexible service
	Meets local population needs
	Fits with national, local and hospital policies
	Creates a service that has long-term survival potential
Weaknesses	Risk of investment in a difficult economic environment
	Recruitment difficulties
	Failure to recapture market share despite increase in capacity
Opportunities	Regain market share
	Repatriate patients
	Capture and create new market segment, e.g. retinal work
Threats	Local competition
	Barriers to entry, e.g. cost of equipment, capacity
	Political climate, e.g. rationalisation of hospitals, or move towards non-hospital based care

SUMMARY

This chapter is an introduction to the increasingly marketised nature of the NHS. It does not attempt to judge whether this is a good or bad change, rather to acknowledge the reality and to enable clinicians to start to develop the language to make the business case, as well as the evidence base, for their service and their patients in this new environment.

By using a case study to examine the changes and how to translate the evidence for change into the business case for change, a framework for clinician involvement in service redesign is identified and explored. An understanding of market principles by clinicians is even more important with the recent shift to GP consortia commissioning. The following chapter looks at finance in more detail.

FURTHER READING

Cooper Z, Gibbons S, Jones S, *et al.* (2010). *Does Hospital Competition Save Lives? Evidence from the recent English NHS choice reforms*. London: LSE. Available at: www2.lse.ac.uk/LSEHealthAndSocialCare/LSEHealth/documents/LSEHealthWorkingPaperSeries.aspx (accessed 20 April 2010).

Cooper ZN, McGuire A, Jones S, *et al.* (2009). Equity, waiting times and NHS reforms: retrospective study. *BMJ*; **339b**: 3274.

Dixon J, editor (March 2010). Proceedings of the Nuffield Trust Annual Health Strategy Summit. Surrey: Nuffield Trust. Available at: www.nuffieldtrust.org.uk/events/detail.aspx?id=46&prID=676&year=2010 (accessed 20 April 2010).

Geisinger Health System. Healthcare reform and Geisenger. www.geisinger.org/about/healthier/index.html

Look After Our NHS. www.lookafterournhs.org.uk/

McCay L, Jonas S (2009). *A Junior Doctor's Guide to the NHS*. London: Medical Directorate Department of Health. Available at: http://group.bmj.com/group/affinity-and-society-publishing/NHS%20Guide.pdf (accessed 20 April 2010).

McKinsey and Company (2002). *Business Plan Preparation: manual for entrepreneurs*. Available at: www.cartierwomensinitiative.com/site/uploads/pdf/McKinsey%20BP%20advice.pdf (accessed 24 June 2010).

NHS Institute for Improvement and Innovation. *Focus on Cataracts*. Warwick: National Institute for Improvement and Innovation; 2008. Available at: www.institute.nhs.uk/index.php?option=com_joomcart&Itemid=194&main_page=document_product_info&cPath=71&products_id=388&Joomcartid=bf4alqdq8qa6rhrpjn80puaij1 (accessed 20 April 2010).

Porter ME (January 2008). The five competitive forces that shape strategy. *Harvard Business Review*; **79**: 79–93.

CHAPTER 9

Basics for the boardroom

Show me the money.

Jerry Maguire

INTRODUCTION

For most doctors, finance is a word uttered in hushed tones: something that falls into the 'managers' domain'. Yet, doctors are the main spenders of NHS resources: organising tests, referring patients, performing procedures. Clear evidence identifies that one of the most powerful mechanisms to reduce spend on potentially unnecessary processes are to identify costs to those ordering the process. Similarly, there is an increasing body of evidence that efficiency and productivity gains can be made if doctors, in particular clinical leads, have control over budgets. To expect doctors to take on these tasks either on a patient basis or a service level is unfair without due training. Yet, all too often that is what happens – few GPs receive 'management training' and yet are all too quickly in the position of managing a small (or indeed sometimes technically medium sized) business.

This chapter is an attempt to provide insight into the rudiments of money matters as they pertain to health. It is not a 'how to' guide to accounting, or a comprehensive analysis of all the issues that affect finance. Rather it is meant to break down the fear barrier and enable readers to investigate further with confidence. This chapter is a starting point for those not currently pursuing management studies. For those in such programmes it is an entry point to translating general learning to the health-care environment.

A ROUGH GUIDE TO THE CURRENT OVERALL PICTURE OF NHS SPENDING

Whilst the aim of this chapter is to allow clinicians to be more willing to become actively involved in the money matters of their own services, it is important to understand a little about where the service fits within the bigger picture.

The budget for the NHS is set as part of the Comprehensive Spending Review, which outlines the spending for three years (the last one in 2007 set spending up to 2011). This is overseen by bi-annual scrutiny of this plan by parliament via the budget and the pre-budget report. As promised by Tony Blair, the current spend on the NHS is roughly in line with the European average, i.e. about 8% of GDP.

The allocated monies are given to the Department of Health who then allocates the revenue expenditure and the capital expenditure (day-to-day spend and large sunk costs respectively). At present this money is then trickled down to the Strategic Health Authorities (SHAs) and Primary Care Trusts (PCTs), and other bodies, e.g. National Patient Safety Agency (NPSA). The vast majority of the spending is via the PCTs. The PCTs receive their proportion of the revenue spending based on a complex formula that is hotly debated. It is an attempt to take into account the local demography, their particular needs and the local effect on salaries, etc. Capital funding comes from a DH pot for which organisations including PCTs and Foundation Trusts (FT) must bid. They are encouraged to use their own funds. In addition, it is also possible to access monies via Private Finance Initiatives (PFI). PFI is a mechanism by which capital projects are financed by non-NHS companies who are repaid over time with annual 'fees'. In the future, GPs, acting in consortia, will play an increasing role commissioning care on behalf of patients.

Whilst NHS organisations are encouraged to ensure that they spend money according to the particular needs of the local population, there are key corporate, i.e. NHS and DH objectives that are identified through the annual Operating Framework.

PCTs are now virtually all commissioners of healthcare (rather than commissioners and providers). This means that it is their responsibility to buy healthcare services from providers, be they NHS, third sector or private. Other options include GPs via Practice Based Commissioning. Whilst PCTs have some ability to negotiate contracts, through service level agreements (SLAs) there are standard 'prices' for some processes, e.g. outpatient visits (new and follow-up), some operations and some hospital admissions. These are designed around categorising the process by the diagnoses (based on a classification called health resource groups (HRGs)), e.g. a hip replacement in an otherwise well under-65-year-old costs XX; if they have additional disease it costs YY. Built into this payment are an expected number of hospital bed days (prolonged stays may allow increased payment). Until recently, this was irrespective of the cause for the prolongation, however as Never Events (inexcusable outcomes) start to develop this is likely to change, and the cost of extensions of stay due to iatrogenic harm will be borne (at least in part) by the hospital. As PCTs had their funding allocation adjusted for the population's make up, so too do hospitals. This means quoted prices are not exactly the numbers that hospitals receive. Similarly, local negotiations with PCTs may set the maximum number of operations paid for. If more are done, these are at the hospital's expense unless new negotiations occur.

As explored in the previous chapter, these prices are defined under the Payment by Results (PbR) and are called the tariff for the process. The price for any given tariff is based at present mainly on the average cost of carrying out the procedure. The problem with this approach is that hospitals have, to date, been poor at costing procedures and do not have figures for each part of the procedure. Most hospitals would struggle to explain how much an X-ray, let alone surgery, really costs. Thus many hospitals are slowly and painfully developing what is known as Activity Based Costing. In essence this is the ability to cost at the individual action level, and requires complex IT and pulling together of multiple data sources.

PbR tariff payments change over time and are a powerful method to allow payment to follow the patient and therefore underpin the 'choice agenda' and influence how care is provided (*see* Chapter 8 for discussion of choice and the market effect). Recently, for example, the tariff has been amended in some areas to only pay for high quality care pathway bundles rather than individual parts of the pathway. The hope is that this will drive providers to create more efficient pathways, e.g. reducing the number of visits to the hospital.

Outpatient appointments work slightly differently. They too are priced based on specialty, but there is less granularity, with divisions for new outpatient appointments and follow ups with variation being possible (if there are multi-professional or multi-disciplinary approaches). Procedures carried out in outpatients are also under the PbR system.

Thus hospitals receive the majority of their funding by 'billing' PCTs for the work they do via SLAs based mainly on the PbR system. However, they do also receive monies directly from the DH, e.g. for teaching, research and other income. Details of the exact sources of money are clarified in the annual accounts/financial statements.

The exact form of the accounts and rules that apply are determined by the status of the organisation, i.e. Foundation Trust (FT). FTs are organisations that in essence have earned increased autonomy as a result of reaching stringent standards as decried by Monitor. For non-FTs there are a few key principles that the trusts must adhere to: breaking even (over a 3-, exceptionally 5-year period) spending on capital must be within set limits and the amount of cash that is available is also set. For FTs they need not break even however they must meet their plan objectives. FTs are monitored against their financial plan by Monitor.

Irrespective of the type of trust, all will have financial plans which lay out expenditure over 3–5 years, supporting the strategic plan of the organisation. The boards of trusts monitor performance against this plan through monthly finance reports, which look at the current position, the near future based on forecasting from the present, and how this compares to where the trust 'should be' according to its plan.

THE BASICS OF ACCOUNTING

Accounting is an ancient art. Monks developed double entry bookkeeping in the medieval period. The aim of accounts is to summarise the financial position of the organisation. Whilst this appears to be a seemingly simple statement, the complications begin as soon as attempts are made to put this principle into practice. A simple example is what constitutes a sale: does it happen the day the order is made, the day it is shipped or the day the order arrives at the purchaser, or even the day the purchaser actually pays for the order (more often than not goods or services are paid in arrears). Thus to try and account for this and create some standardisation, accounting rules and principles have been developed. In addition to country, regional or industry regulation there are standards and guidelines known as the Generally Accepted Accounting Principles (GAAP), which attempt to provide guidance on how best to deal with accounting situations – however they are not mandatory. Each company therefore starts its accounts by explaining its policy (the combination of the laws and practices it follows). This is further clarified by a system of notes that are used to accompany financial information to try and explain the rationale behind the accounting practice. The net result though of such practices is to force the user to understand that accounts cannot be viewed as absolute; they are a subjective analysis of the financial situation.

NHS accounts must follow 'industry standards' as defined by the Secretary of State or Monitor, over and above the legal requirements for the UK. These state that there must be four sections to the accounts: the balance sheet, the profit and loss (P and L) or income and expenditure account, the cash flow statement and a statement of total gains and losses at an organisation level. To ensure that the accounts are acceptable, there is an internal audit committee who reviews the accounts before they are put to the board, and accounts are audited (looked at) by external auditors.

Four key principles that underpin accounts are: accruals, prudence, consistency and viability. The concept of accruals means that a transaction is recorded as having occurred at the moment that the transaction is made, rather than when payment occurs. Prudence and consistency focus on the need to use conservative estimates and to do so consistently (if changes to practice are made they must be clearly identified). Viability is the concept that an organisation will continue to exist.

THE BALANCE SHEET

The balance sheet is a summary of where the organisation is at in terms of its finances (*see* Box 9.1 for an example from St Anywhere). It includes all the parts of the organisation that could be deemed as 'assets', i.e. something of value, and all of the liabilities, i.e. monies owed.

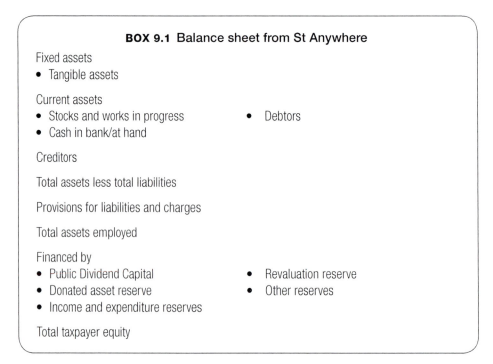

BOX 9.1 Balance sheet from St Anywhere

Fixed assets
• Tangible assets

Current assets
• Stocks and works in progress   • Debtors
• Cash in bank/at hand

Creditors

Total assets less total liabilities

Provisions for liabilities and charges

Total assets employed

Financed by
• Public Dividend Capital   • Revaluation reserve
• Donated asset reserve   • Other reserves
• Income and expenditure reserves

Total taxpayer equity

Assets may be broken down into fixed assets (long-term assets), e.g. an MRI scanner, and current (short-term assets), e.g. cash. Within the fixed asset category are three subsections: tangible assets – physical assets; intangible assets, i.e. something the organisation possesses but is not physical such as intellectual property or patents; and investments, e.g. shares in another organisation that will not be sold within the next 12 months. These last two categories are of less use in the NHS. Current assets consist of stock held, i.e. inventory which can be sub-grouped as raw materials, work in progress and finished goods (stocks might for example be pharmacy stock); debtors, i.e. those who owe the organisation money, other (which includes items like tax rebates) and cash.

The liabilities section consists of current (short-term) and long-term. The short-term is subdivided into: creditors (monies owed to other organisations); tax payable; leases; accruals (monies owed for bills, e.g. utilities); short-term debt, e.g. overdrafts; and of less importance in the NHS, dividends payable. Long-term liabilities are bank loans, e.g. mortgages.

The balance sheet then summarises the position, i.e. total assets minus total liabilities. The final section of a non-NHS balance sheet would include how this money is divided up. In the case of the NHS, all of this is called tax-payers' equity.

THE INCOME AND EXPENDITURE STATEMENT OR PROFIT AND LOSS STATEMENTS

This is in essence the summary of where the organisation is at overall – i.e. how much it has spent and earned, rather than what it holds and what it owes. *See* Box 9.2 for an example from St Anywhere.

BOX 9.2 Income and expenditure for St Anywhere 2008

- Income from activities
- Other operating income
- Operating expenses
- OPERATING SURPLUS/ DEFICIT
- Profit on disposal of fixed assets
- Interest receivable
- Surplus or deficit before interest (operating profit)
- Interest payable
- SURPLUS/ DEFICIT FOR THE YEAR
- Public Dividend Capital Dividend Repayable for the Year
- RETAINED SURPLUS/DEFICIT FOR THE YEAR

The Income and Expenditure statement (I+E) is read downwards. For non-NHS companies, the first line is generally sales, followed by the cost of sales thereby generating the gross profit. The next section concerns operating expenses. For the NHS, first, there is the income generated over the year, which may be broken into: the income from activities (seeing patients), and other operating income. The operating expenses may then be delineated. Thus the operating profit (or loss) can be identified, i.e. the income minus the expenses. Added to this is any monies raised from selling off fixed assets, thereby giving the next line, i.e. the surplus or deficit before interest, which would be known in non-NHS terms as the operating profit or the earnings before interest tax depreciation and amortisation (the infamous EBITDA). Depreciation and amortisation are technical ways for dealing with value changes over time.

The next section is about the interest payable. Once this is taken into account, alongside any exceptional costs, the surplus or deficit for the year is created (in non-NHS terminology, the profit before tax). Accounts then have the tax liable on the previous amount and hence the profit after tax. Finally, any dividends payable are taken into account and what is left is the retained profit. Since the NHS does not pay tax, instead the public dividend and capital dividends payable are taken off, leaving the retained surplus or deficit.

CASHFLOW STATEMENT

BOX 9.3 Cashflow statement for St Anywhere

- OPERATING ACTIVITIES
- Net cash inflow/(outflow) from operating activities
- RETURNS ON INVESTMENTS AND SERVICING OF FINANCE
- Interest received
- Interest paid
- Net cash inflow from returns on investments and servicing of finance
- CAPITAL EXPENDITURE AND FINANCIAL INVESTMENT
- Payments to acquire tangible fixed assets
- Receipts from sale of tangible fixed assets
- Net cash outflow from capital expenditure
- DIVIDENDS PAID
- Net cash inflow/(outflow) before management of liquid resources and financing
- MANAGEMENT OF LIQUID RESOURCES
- Sale of investments
- Net cash inflow from management of liquid resources
- Net cash inflow/(outflow) before financing
- FINANCING
- Public dividend capital repaid (not previously accrued)
- Other capital receipts
- Net cash inflow/(outflow) from financing
- Increase/(decrease) in cash

The cashflow statement explains how the monies are managed, e.g. how the finance department is ensuring that there is sufficient cash for salaries, etc. but are not leaving too much money in low interest accounts to facilitate this. The cashflow allows understanding of the day-to-day management prowess of the organisation.

Essentially the cashflow is divided into blocks: normal expenditure, interest and dividends, taxes (less relevant), investment activity and financing. Ultimately working through the cash flow statement line by line, allows you to ascertain the amount of cash available after all the additions and deductions have occurred. Cash is king and this gives an inkling of management abilities.

The final mandatory report is recognised gains and losses, which acts as a companion to the cashflow statement and focuses on shifts in money from a baseline, thereby giving a bird's eye view of financial health.

BOX 9.4 St Anywhere recognised gains and losses

- Surplus for the financial year before dividend payments
- Unrealised surplus/(deficit) on fixed asset revaluations/indexation
- Increases in the donated asset reserve due to receipt of donated financed assets
- Reductions in the donated asset reserve due to the depreciation and disposal of donated assets
- Total gains and losses recognised in the financial period

MAKING SENSE OF THE NUMBERS

Whilst the reports themselves are important statements, much more information can be gleaned by detailed analysis of the reports. As with other fields like biostatistics, which whilst seemingly mathematically based have a considerable degree of subjectivity (and even philosophy), traditions have developed that enable these deductions to be comparable. The key tradition is using ratios. Essentially this just means putting one number over another. In the business world, key ratios cover a variety of areas. One often talked about example is ROCE (the return on capital employed). This is calculated by dividing operating profit by the shareholders' funds and long-term liabilities. This gives potential investors a clue as to how much money they might get back (ideally more than they could get anywhere else, such as the bank!). This also provides information about the viability of the business. If the ROCE is not higher than interest rates, the company will be paying out more (in interest repayments) than it makes on any monies that it has taken out as loans.

IS MONEY EVERYTHING?

So far this chapter has rightly focused on the money. But clearly money is not everything, as a number of recent investigations, most pointedly Mid Staffordshire, identified. In fact, when this hospital in particular focused too much on finance, patient care and healthcare quality dropped to unimaginably low levels. Businesses, and indeed other public sector organisations, have started to balance this by using a technique known as a balance scorecard. This is, in essence, methodology to try and provide equal weights to other aspects of hospitals and organisations' output thereby ensuring that too much attention is not focused on one domain. The non-finance elements are the customer, internal business processes, and learning and growth. Whilst many do not use these categories rigorously, the benefit of the approach derives not just from the countermeasures to finance but also because it forces organisations to identify (and sometimes rank) what matters. Furthermore, it means that similar metrics can be used at a divisional level and then aggregated to an institutional level. This is because to really work, a scorecard needs to be additive, e.g. the same or similar metrics need to apply throughout the organisation. The operating framework and using the vital signs alongside quality accounts are examples of how NHS thinking has developed along these lines.

SUMMARY

This chapter has attempted to show the broad financial landscape in which organisations sit. Furthermore, the key financial documents of the NHS are explored, and how these relate to non-NHS accounting practices. The chapter also looks at how organisations and indeed the NHS are trying to cope with balancing the importance of finance with other measures such as healthcare quality.

FURTHER READING

Atril P, McLaney E (2007). *Management Accounting for Decision Makers.* 5th ed. Harlow: Pearson Education Limited.

Audit Commission (2009). *A Guide to Finance for NHS Doctors.* London: Academy of Medical Royal Colleges. Available at: www.auditcommission.gov.uk/health/audit/financial mgmt/hospitaldoctors/Pages/hospitaldoctors9jul2009.aspx#downloads (accessed 20 April 2010).

Brookson S (2010). *Essential Managers: understanding accounts.* Hampton: Dorling Kindersley.

Castro PJ, Dorgan SJ, Richardson B (February 2008). A healthier healthcare system for the UK. *McKinsey Quarterly.* Available at: www.mckinseyquarterly.com/A_healthier_health_care_system_for_the_United_Kingdom_2101 (accessed 20 April 2010).

Department of Health (2009). *Payment by Results 2010–11 Road Test Package.* London: Department of Health. Available at: www.dh.gov.uk/en/Publicationsandstatistics/Publications/PublicationsPolicyAndGuidance/DH_110106 (accessed 20 April 2010).

Department of Health (2010) *NHS Operating Framework 2010–11.* London: Department of Health. Available at: www.dh.gov.uk/en/Publicationsandstatistics/Publications/Publications PolicyAndGuidance/DH_110107 (accessed 20 April 2010).

Department of Health (2010). *Robert Francis Inquiry Report into Mid-Staffordshire NHS Foundation Trust.* London: Department of Health. Available at: www.dh.gov.uk/en/Publications andstatistics/Publications/PublicationsPolicyAndGuidance/DH_113018 (accessed 20 April 2010).

Kaplan R, Norton D (January–February 1992). The balanced scorecard: measures that drive performance. *Harvard Business Review;* 70–9.

Lebas MJ, Stolowy H (2006). *Financial Accounting and Reporting.* 2nd ed. London: Thomson Learning.

Monitor: Independent Regulator of NHS Foundation Trusts. Service-line management. Available at: www.monitor-nhsft.gov.uk/home/developing-nhs-foundation-trusts/service-line-management-0

Mountford J, Webb C (2008). *Clinical Leadership: unlocking high performance in healthcare.* London: McKinsey and Company.

National Patient Safety Agency (2010). *Never Events Framework Update for 2010–11.* London: National Patient Safety Agency. Available at: www.nrls.npsa.nhs.uk/resources/?entryid45= 68518&char=N (accessed 20 April 2010).

Nevers RL (December 2002). A financial argument for service-line management. *Healthcare Financial Management*; **56**(12): 38–42.

Patel KCR, Spilsbury P (2010). The UK National Health Service approach to the economic crisis. *J R Soc Med*; **103**: 123–4.

Quattrone P (2004). Accounting for God: accounting and accountability practices in the Society of Jesus (Italy, XVI-XVII centuries). *Accounting, Organizations and Society Volume*; **29**(7): 647–83.

Rosen R, Corrigan P, Appleby J, *et al.* (2010). Can the NHS cut costs without substantially damaging the quality of health care? *BMJ*; **340**: 835–7.

CHAPTER 10

Marketing speak

Many a small thing has been made large by the right kind of advertising.

Mark Twain

INTRODUCTION

If you are misfortunate enough to have an ill child, there is some comfort in knowing they are being treated in the best possible place. The name 'Great Ormond Street Hospital' instills confidence in many parents of unwell children. The name also carries kudos on many aspiring trainees' curriculum vitae. However, most paediatricians would agree that while Great Ormond Street undoubtedly has some great departments and inspirational clinicians and researchers, it is by no means the best place for all aspects of healthcare, despite its amazingly strong public reputation and brand.

If brands matter for clothes, food and handbags, surely they matter too for healthcare. Or, do the values of the NHS bypass the power and influence of branding and marketing? The NHS itself is an incredibly strong brand. Not only the largest employer in the country but the fourth largest in the world, behind only the Chinese Army, the Indian Railway and Wal-Mart!

Experience in the US has demonstrated that if healthcare is left to the free market, this can lead to over treatment (Gawande, 2009). Despite the principles of equality that underpin the NHS, there are undoubtedly certain brands within the NHS such as 'The Brompton' and 'The Marsden' that are internationally recognisable. These brands convey what is known as a value proposition. This, and other marketing concepts and tools, will be discussed in this chapter with relevance to healthcare.

Marketing for health does not solely relate to the healthcare organisation's communication to potential patients or customers. The concept of internal marketing refers to how employees are trained to provide optimal customer service or patient experience. The Chartered Institute of Marketing defines marketing as 'the management process responsible for identifying, anticipating and satisfying customer requirements profitably' (CIM, 2010). This means identifying target markets and satisfying these customers. There is more to marketing than advertising alone. Chapter 8 considered how ophthalmology services could be most effectively marketed to both GPs and patients, to support the business case.

It is impossible to predict the future. However, with increasing overlap between private and public healthcare sectors, doctors may follow the model of barristers and deliver healthcare from chambers instead of hospitals. The 'choose and book' system is a step towards this. If this market evolves further, doctors would need to learn how to attract patients rather than expecting patients to automatically arrive as passive customers irrespective of clinical performance and ability. At present, doctors receive a relatively secure and comfortable salary, without the need to actively attract patients. It seems likely that future models of care delivery will bring the worlds of marketing and medicine closer together. Already, some GPs' salaries are linked to measures of patient experience.

Web innovations such as iwantgreatcare.com have taken advantage of the need to openly disclose feedback on clinician performance to patients, and the opportunity to harness the power of the internet:

> It took just 40 years for the first 50 million people to own a radio; just 16 years for the first 50 million people to own a PC; but just 5 years for the first 50 million to be on the Internet.
>
> (HM Treasury, 2007)

Since the World Wide Web first emerged in 1990, the impact of technology on social networks has been profound. Information about healthcare and performance is more widely, cheaply and immediately accessible than ever and can be used to attract patients. Already, patients are able to choose their GP and where they want to be treated. This chapter will unpack how marketing tools can be used to navigate the healthcare market.

Marketing speak is similar to medical speak. It is another language full of acronyms and conceptual frameworks. This chapter aims to translate some of these unfamiliar models into digestible sections, with applicability to healthcare. It also introduces the concept of the personal brand and self-marketing.

Whilst examples of marketing often relate to specific products, the principles are equally applicable to services such as healthcare. A service is defined as an intangible product involving performance that cannot physically be possessed. Other examples include education, tourism and finance. The key differentiating characteristics of services from products are: intangibility, inseparability of production and consumption, perishability, client-based relationships and customer contact.

BACKGROUND

One of the most popular and straightforward marketing tools is the PEST analysis. This analyses the Political, Environmental, Social and Technological environment. Box 10.1 shows a PEST analysis of the British healthcare environment (as of April, 2010). It is not an all-inclusive analysis but provides a context to understand the key drivers for change. As well as an essential ingredient for business plans, a PEST analysis is also a useful framework for responding to interview or essay questions on current changes in healthcare!

BOX 10.1 PEST analysis

Political

Changes in government inevitably lead to potentially radical shifts in healthcare policies. At present these include the future prospect of an independent NHS with further reorganisation and the blurring of boundaries between the NHS and the independent sector.

Increasing shift of healthcare delivery into the community:

- Vertical integration linking primary and secondary care
- Closer working relationship between health and social care.

Since 2009, the European Working Time Directive (EWTD) has limited the working hours of doctors in training to 48 hours per week. This has reduced the time available for training and experiential learning. In part, this has been compensated for with an increased consultant workload.

There has been a shift from a target driven culture to a regulated culture, with local control of measures of success.

The British Medical Association (BMA) is a powerful union with an increasing political stance, e.g. 'Keep NHS public campaign' (2010).

Economic

The current financially ischaemic status of the NHS demands substantial increases in clinical productivity and efficiency.

Following the introduction of EWTD, wherever possible, tasks that have traditionally been carried out by doctors are given to non-medical healthcare teams. Evidence suggests that this is not always a more cost-effective approach.

Rather than GPs acting as gatekeepers to specialist NHS services, GPs increasingly act as providers of services, including minor procedures, delivering care closer to the patient's home.

There is increasing acceptance of the healthcare service as a business at all levels of the NHS.

Social

The social demographics of the British population are changing, alongside growing expectations of patients, increasing prevalence of long-term conditions (over 15 million), increasing life expectancy of individuals with multiple health problems and widening health inequalities.

In addition to population changes, the needs and expectations of medical trainees are evolving, including shifts in gender demographics, increasing pursuit of a good work-life balance and improved support networks.

The introduction of EWTD has led to the breakdown of the traditional 'clinical firm' model of medicine. The shift patterns of trainees and their consultant trainers coincide less often, providing less opportunity for trainees to follow their patients through.

Generation Y (those born between 1980 and mid-1990s) are much less likely to stay in a job-for-life (James, 2008). A challenge for the NHS is that this generation is more likely to take time out for personal life enhancement and demand a flexible working environment with immediate rewards for hard work.

Although polls consistently demonstrate that the wider population considers doctors the most trusted profession, the social context in which patients interact with doctors has changed in several ways. For example, levels of education and overall earnings among the population are increasing. Alongside this, the internet has broadened access to globalised healthcare markets and research. This has led to rising expectations of what the NHS should provide and deliver.

Social relations are becoming more fluid and less hierarchical with less deference towards authority and a greater drive towards individualism. The public is becoming more autonomous and questioning yet by contrast, traditional hierarchies within the medical profession persist.

Technological

The use of social networking channels including twitter.com, facebook.com and linkedin.com offer potential viral marketing opportunities to engage with clinical communities.

The antiquated one-way communication of bleeps has been replaced by iPhone apps in some hospitals (iBleep, Salford Royal).

Education and teaching are increasingly streamed as online modules.

The construct of virtual wards blurs the boundaries between primary and secondary care (Croydon Primary Care Trust).

Electronic Health Records aim to help prevent error and improve service co-ordination. Crucially, they offer an opportunity to engage clinicians with aggregate patient data sets.

E-handover, as in Sheffield hospital, aims to reduce the human error associated with attempting to remember individual patient details or scribbling comments on pieces of paper.

Developments in surgical technology, such as laporoscopic procedures, have reduced patient recovery time and led to the creation of new disciplines such as Intervention Radiology (IR).

Bedside dashboards, under development at Imperial Business School, London, collate predictive models for clinical situations with costing data and population level information.

Imperial College and the London Deanery have pioneered the role of simulation for health professionals. Portable simulation operating theatres facilitate widened access to this learning opportunity (DH, 2008).

MARKETING MIX

The guiding principles for marketing are orientated around the customer, or patient. Creating a marketing strategy involves selecting marketing opportunities to pursue, and analysing a target market to create an appropriate marketing mix.

The marketing mix can sometimes be described as the '5 Ps': product, place/ distribution, promotion, price and people. All aspects of the marketing mix aim to meet the needs of the consumer, or patient.

Product

For the NHS, the product being provided is a service for healthcare, e.g. the opthalmology service described in Chapter 8. The same principles of marketing apply to a service as for a product. For the NHS, the nature of the service may be a consultation, a prescription, a procedure such as an operation or advice about prevention.

Place

Healthcare is traditionally provided by GP surgeries and hospitals. More recently, Private Finance Initiatives and Independent Sector Treatment Centres have entered the market. The aim of marketing is to satisfy customers. This means providing the right service at the right time in a convenient location. Increasingly, care is being provided out of and away from hospitals. Improving customer experience has led to lengthened GP opening hours. There is a rapidly growing market of e-health initiatives, through online communities seeking to provide alternative and/or additional support and information for patients.

Promotion

Promotion or 'marketing communications', means communication about NHS activities and services to the local population. This can be done through a variety of communication channels, including posters, directly mailing leaflets and using the internet to advertise or email patients. The NHS has a lot to learn from the expertise of marketeers in delivering messages in a personalised way to match individual ethnic origin, income, employment, age, interests and other key characteristics.

Price

In any market, the price of the product determines how consumers perceive it. The unique underlying principle for the NHS is that healthcare is free at the point of use and available to everyone based on need, not ability to pay. The possibility exists that individuals value healthcare more when they pay for it, for example, from a private provider. Applying this principle, some GP clinics have successfully reduced non-attendance rates by charging people if they do not attend, therein attaching value to the service.

People

In healthcare, the people aspect of the marketing mix is for those delivering frontline care. It also includes people who are involved in other aspects of the marketing mix. All of these are crucial to developing a successful marketing strategy.

If we look to St Anywhere and their attempt to market their midwifery led unit, the benefit of this approach becomes clear. Whilst St Anywhere may not directly market to patients, it could, for example, reach GPs through a series of lectures on obstetrics, presented by the St Anywhere Professor of Obstetrics.

MARKETING TOOLS AND TECHNIQUES

Shared decision-making aids in healthcare use marketing know-how to empower and inform the patient. These tools aim to support people to understand the likely outcomes of options they face for treatment and to consider their personal values as they relate to the risks and benefits of each option. Decision aids may be DVDs, workbooks or websites. They are particularly useful when there is no clear 'best' treatment option. At present, they are under-utilised in the NHS. A good example of where shared decision-making has been embedded into patient care pathways can be found at the Dartmouth-Hitchcock Medical Centre, USA. There, surgeons will not discuss treatment options with patients until they have visited the shared decision-making centre to research their choices.

Most marketing plans would be incomplete without including a SWOT analysis, as seen in Chapter 9. This simple approach identifies strengths (S) on which to build, weaknesses (W) to rectify, opportunities (O) to consider and threats (T) to address. Whilst individuals or teams can rapidly create SWOTs, they are most effective if the lists under each of the four sections are ranked in order of importance, evidence-based and specific, rather than vague and not too long! Strengths and weaknesses tend to refer to internal factors, whereas opportunities and threats tend to be external. Table 9.1 shows an example of a SWOT analysis.

The Ansoff matrix is another popular marketing tool, shown in Figure 10.1, to assist marketing decision-making.

Market penetration is about increasing sales in current markets with current products and services. Whilst this is less important for the NHS, market penetration for new entrants to the healthcare market such as Independent Sector Treatment Centres (ISTCs), penetration is the main goal and overcoming the barriers to entry discussed in Chapter 8.

Market development is increasing sales of current products and services in new markets. An example of this is thinking about how the NHS could export some of its services and skills to the international healthcare market.

Product/service development occurs through increasing sales by improving present products or developing new products for current markets, as per example of the opthalmology service in St Anywhere Hospital in Chapter 9. In the NHS, over the last two years, several GP surgeries have evolved into polyclinics offering a wider range of healthcare services including minor operations.

Market	Product	**Present**	**New**
Present		Market penetration	Product development
New		Market development	Diversification

FIGURE 10.1 Ansoff's competitive strategies

Source: Ansoff HI (1988). *The New Corporate Strategy.* New York: John Wiley and Sons.

Diversified growth occurs when new products are developed and sold in new markets. An example of this in health is the creation of some of the new Masters in Medical Leadership by UK universities, Section 1, being simultaneously taught in Singapore and Asia. These courses are both new products and are reaching new markets.

SEGMENTATION

Segmentation is the grouping of customers into smaller, homogeneous segments with similar requirements and characteristics. This can be done in many ways including geographically, by age and by condition. This segmentation approach can then be used to risk-stratify patient populations, for example, according to their risk of requiring hospital admission. Once segments have been identified, marketing of specific and appropriate services can then be tailored to that segment.

Segmentation can also be used to understand the complexities of the UK healthcare ecosystem, shown by the above PEST analysis. For example, it may be helpful to group the key organisations in healthcare into groups, shown in Box 10.2.

BOX 10.2 Stakeholders in the UK healthcare system

- Professional bodies, such as the Royal Colleges.
- Employers, such as NHS Trusts and Primary Care Trusts (PCTs).
- Regulators, such as Care Quality Commission (CQC) and Monitor.
- Educational bodies, such as Medical Education England (MEE).
- Academic service collaborations, such as Academic Health Sciences Centres.
- Policy makers and the Department of Health. This includes think tanks such as the Nuffield Trust and the King's Fund.
- Patient organisations, such as the Patients Association and Patient Voices.
- International improvement bodies, such as the Institute for Healthcare Improvement (IHI).
- Independent healthcare organisations, such as Bupa, Care UK and Circle. These organisations are playing an increasing role in cannibalising the NHS monopoly and influencing the evolution of UK healthcare provision. Despite its opponents, competition of provision is likely to improve the quality of healthcare.

Box 10.2 is not exhaustive but provides a framework for considering the UK healthcare economy in segments.

SELF-MARKETING

This chapter has mainly focused on marketing for organisations. One of the imprints that an MBA imparts on individuals is a sense of self-confidence and the ability to self-market. This is sometimes called 'personal branding'. This skill is especially important for medics who may be embarking on a career transition, as many who do MBAs will be. Being confident about your distinctive strengths, through conducting a self-SWOT analysis will hold you in a strong position despite any uncertainty you may feel about next career steps. Chapters 15 and 16 include an overview of potential career paths for medics with MBAs.

SUMMARY

As an organisation, the NHS is committed towards becoming a more patient-centric service. Marketing offers a mechanism for enhancing consumer awareness. As such, it matters as much for the NHS and healthcare in general as for any business.

There is much that the NHS could learn from the corporate sector about enhancing customer service and experience. Measuring how well customers' expectations are being met is crucial: individually, through surveys and in focus groups. Some data on patient experience is now being routinely collected as PROMs (Patient Reported Outcome Measures) for a minority of procedures.

Effective marketing has been directly linked to improvements in business performance. Given the potential for marketing techniques to directly improve the quality of care delivered by healthcare providers and commissioners, we question how long it will be before the Department of Health appoints a Director General for Marketing.

FURTHER READING

Appleby J, Crawford R, Emmerson C (2009). How cold will it be? *Prospects for NHS Funding 2011–2017*. London: The King's Fund.

Department of Health (2008). *Chief Medical Officer's Annual Report*. Safer medical practice: machines, manikins and polo mints. London: Department of Health.

Dibb S, Simkin L, Pride WM, *et al.* (2006). *Marketing Concepts and Strategies*. Boston: Houghton Mifflin.

Earls M (2009). *Herd: how to change mass behaviour by harnessing our true behaviour*. Chichester: John Wiley & Sons, Ltd.

Ferrell OC, Dibb S, Simkin L, *et al.* (2005). *Marketing: concepts and strategies*. 5th ed. Boston: Houghton Mifflin (Academic).

Flannery P (2007). Look for the similarities. *Quirk's Marketing Research Review*.

Gawande A (June 2009). The cost conundrum. *The New Yorker*.

iBleep. www.ibleep.net

James J, Bibb S, Walker S (2008). *Generation Y: what they want from work*. A summary report of the 'Tell it how it is' research. London: Talentsmoothie. Available at: www.talentsmoothie. com/wp-content/uploads/2009/12/TIHIS-report-Summary-and-Conclusion.pdf (accessed 18 June 2010).

Pathiraja F, Taylor J (2010). Branding your career. *BMJ Careers*.

Postgraduate Medical Education and Training Board (PMETB) (2008). *Educating Tomorrow's Doctors: future models of medical training. Medical workforce shape and trainee expectations*. London: PMETB.

The Chartered Institute of Marketing. www.cim.co.uk

Woolfson T (2010). Marketing and Medicine. *BMJ Careers*.

CHAPTER 11

Inch pebbles and nudges: management of change

If we want things to stay as they are, they will have to change.

Giuseppe Tomasi di Lampedusa, The Leopard

INTRODUCTION

Healthcare has a clear dichotomy: on the one hand clinicians are often enormously excited about innovation and research developments; on the other they are very hesitant about making changes to practice. For many clinicians the desire to be at the forefront of scientific research is part of the challenge and excitement of medicine. Yet, we see all too often how slow and difficult it can be to implement the changes that are often the corollaries of these efforts. Coupled with this is the political landscape of healthcare in the UK. The fact that the NHS is a publicly funded system means that responsibility rests ultimately with politicians. The complicated needs of the political system mean that the healthcare environment is often vulnerable to repeated cycles of change, especially structural change. Thus, staying still is not an option.

MAKING CHANGE HAPPEN

Change management, as a subject, is all encompassing; core to business teaching, yet absent from medical curricula. It covers everything from how to alter individual personal traits through to how to alter the direction of huge conglomerates. The literature surrounding change management is vast. This chapter is not an academic evaluation of change management, rather it is intended to give a few insights into the concepts and the key ideas that are in vogue at present. In particular, through extending the example of St Anywhere and applying popular concepts of behavioural economics, it is hoped that it inspires clinicians who are rightly sceptical of change to be slightly less cautious.

A key source of resistance for change in healthcare is 'investment lock-in'; a significant portion of the NHS budget is already allocated for specific services. In addition, the dispersal of power throughout the NHS means that a revolutionary process of change may not be possible and an evolutionary approach is more likely.

An evolutionary approach involves constant moderate changes accumulated over a long period to produce a large cumulative result. This is likely to take years. The punctuated equilibrium model of change describes long periods of small, incremental change interrupted by brief periods of discontinuous change. This means that periods of upheaval and turmoil are brief and a new equilibrium is established during the periods of stability. Healthcare professionals in the NHS are often heard complaining about continual change – 'change fatigue'. This resistance to change by NHS employees is in conflict with the contemporary view that organisations change 'continuously'. Examples from industry show that the continued success of a change effort depends on succeeding that effort with continued change.

The doyen of change management is Kotter. Through studying thousands of cases and immersing himself in change programmes, he has developed keen insights into what works and why, in a business setting. His eight points to enable successful change are shown in Box 11.1. Kotter observed that for change to take place, over 75 per cent of the company has to be convinced that business-as-usual is totally unacceptable. This threshold is unlikely to be achieved in the NHS, owing to the number of bystanders and isolates (Chapter 7).

What works in one environment, such as aviation or manufacturing, may not be as successful if directly transposed into another environment, such as healthcare. How the quality improvement methodology or change itself is introduced can often determine the success of the intervention as much as what the intervention itself is. For example, the type of change required for patient safety to become a priority in healthcare is strategic rather than incremental.

BOX 11.1 Kotter's eight critical steps for companies to make a change

1 Creating a sense of urgency for change has to come from the top.
2 Establishing a coalition of the willing is a powerful lever for change outside the normal hierarchy.
3 Developing a vision for where an organisation is trying to go focuses employees on the task at hand.
4 Failure to communicate the vision ultimately halts progress.
5 Removing significant barriers to progress fosters a culture of change.
6 Short-term wins are necessary to keep up momentum.
7 Not being satisfied with small short-term successes and thinking big leads to sustainable long-term change.
8 Ingraining a culture of the way things are done around here is the ultimate test of successful change.

Source: Kotter J (1995). Leading change: why transformation efforts fail. *Harvard Business Review*.

Behavioural economics is the area of economics that overlaps with psychology. It seeks to explain the seemingly irrational behaviour of individuals who fail to act in ways that economic models might otherwise predict. This field is synonymous, perhaps unfortunately, with American single word book titles including *Nudge, Sway* and *Connected*. Whilst this could be considered a fad, the messages of these books are important because they attempt to look holistically at motivations of people and organisations. In particular, they are a useful compliment to the approach of Kotter because they are adapted to environments and cultures where motives are generally intrinsic, i.e. driven by a need for self-fulfilment rather than extrinsically motivated by goals or rewards.

The Mayo Clinic is regularly amongst the top hospitals in the USA in various listings. 'The Mayo' has repeatedly undergone change: through rapid expansion and moves into community-based care, internet-based information and resource development. These changes have occurred precisely because those leading the change understood the motivations of those involved. These change programmes have worked with the culture of the organisation, which is a very strong intrinsically motivated one, rather than imposing change. Dan Ariely, in his book *Predictably Irrational*, devotes a chapter to norms, in which he articulates the difference between market norms and social norms. Market norms are his term for the mechanisms at play in trades for money; social norms the mechanisms at play in non-financial interactions. One of Ariely's examples of social norms is bringing flowers to a dinner party, whereas the market norm – less socially acceptable – would be to offer payment for your share of the meal.

Through a series of experiments on unfortunate college students (often MBA students), Ariely identifies that if market and social norms collide or are blended, social norms shrink. He took three groups of people: one was asked to do a set of tasks out of the goodness of their hearts, one paid minimally and the third group paid slightly more; those doing the tasks for free scored the highest, followed by those who were paid the most, with those paid the least scoring the least. Through this simple experiment, Ariely identifies the power of intrinsic motivation: once extrinsic rewards creep in, behaviour adapts to the reward.

In a similar set of experiments using gifts of different values, there was practically no difference between the scores. When the gift prices were declared, the previously demonstrated extrinsic patterns re-emerged. Ariely goes on to describe an infamous experiment in an Israeli day-care centre, where plagued by parents picking up kids habitually late, fines were introduced. Rather than this solving the problem, the problem got worse: the norms were changed from social to market, and worse still, even after the removal of the fine, the behaviour continued.

It may be worth considering recent reforms in the NHS in this light as an example of how important behavioural economics is to change management. Increasing pay for clinicians, particularly where it has been based on reaching performance goals, has indeed led to improved performance in those goals (although there is much argument about gaming and whether the correct metrics where picked. However, in the main reforms, such as the QOF – Quality of Outcomes Framework – have driven change). The bigger question though is at what price? Have we switched social norms of medicine to market norms and can we ever go back? This is a pertinent question given the current financial crisis. Could we have succeeded in achieving the same effects by using some sort of gift (maintaining social norms) rather than using financial incentives?

For the NHS, this is fundamental and maybe the lesson comes at a key moment. From the NHS plan (2000), accompanying the increase in spend on health was a requirement to show clear results. The mechanisms of performance management were around setting targets, e.g. the 4 hour wait, providing tools to assist in the change and then rigorously patrolling and driving the change. In many ways, this approach created radical change in what had been a relatively inertia-prone environment, due to the large numbers of employees acting as bystanders (Chapter 7). It is hard now walking through accident and emergency departments to remember what it was like when patients used to bring sandwiches to survive lengthy trolley waits. This improvement has come at a price. The price has been a palpable decline in morale, despite increasing pay for clinicians. This was perhaps compounded by the second phase of reform – the phase of financial probity. The NSR (2008) articulated a third stage: one in which clinicians are front and centre, and the emphasis now is on the clinical quality of care. It is within this phase that the perfect dynamic is set up to use the lessons of Kotter and behavioural economics to think about future change. To date, there has been a realisation that to really create a high quality healthcare system along the lines of, for example, the Mayo Clinic, we need people to want to go the extra mile. The lessons to take on board are that this cannot be encouraged by finance alone.

LESSONS FROM KOTTER AND BEHAVIOURAL ECONOMICS

Kotter's steps to transformational change are business focused (Box 11.1), although elements are highly applicable to the public sector. The challenge in transferring and translating comes back to Ariely's core point alluded to earlier, about how you motivate. For Kotter, a fundamental requirement for a successful change programme is to 'create a burning platform'. As Chip and Dan Heath point out in their recent book *Switch* (which is a highly practical guide to change), this analogy comes from the infamous Piper Alpha disaster, where individuals were forced to break norms and change to save their lives; the choice was to stay on board the burning platform or leap into the unknown freezing sea with a burning layer of oil at the surface. Those who jumped survived in higher numbers. Dan Ariely uses a different, although equally extreme, example of Chinese Commander in 210 BC Xiang Yu who burnt his own troops' ships and cooking pots to galvanise them to win. In common parlance we often talk about 'burning bridges' as a method of describing closing off a route back to something. The problem the Heath brothers point out with using this negative language, is similar to that of Ariely: negative motivators can only get you so far, better they argue to motivate using positive methods; they call it 'finding the feeling'.

One such example is that of the creation of a game called Re-Mission. This computer game is aimed at teenage cancer patients undergoing chemotherapy, who chase around a virtual blood stream zapping cancer cells; accompanying this are short infomercials from a robot about chemotherapy and cancer, in between game levels. The game was designed to try and combat poor compliance with medication post-discharge from hospital-based chemotherapy, thereby threatening survival considerably. Amazingly, the game increased chemotherapy blood levels by 20%, thereby doubling the survival rates of the affected adolescents, irrespective of the number of levels of the game played. It wasn't so much the information that was making the difference; it was that the team who developed the game had found a way to motivate the teenagers through their emotions.

As both Kotter and the Heath brothers agree, the key to change is not about finding an analytical solution to the problem and motivating this way. Rather it is about capturing the emotion positively or negatively and allowing this to be the motivator that drives change. Nearly all of the behavioural economics books talk at some level about the division between what some call the rational and the emotional. Whilst the biology might be hard to rationalise, the concept of these two domains is a well-recognised psychological principle.

If the Heaths' and Kotter's prescription for successful change are analysed and compared, the results offer a surprising degree of overlap, shown in Table 11.1. In *Switch*, the Heaths clearly identify which mechanisms connect to the emotional and which to the rational, the benefit being that for those areas where the rational is perhaps more dominant these strategies can be focused on; likewise where it is the emotional these can be focused on. The Heaths add a third domain: the path of change. Kotter too alludes to this but again without delineating those mechanisms that drive this.

However, there are differences: the Heaths start further back in the process by identifying successful change stories (ideally from locally to the change environment about what and who are the bright spots). Equally as mentioned, the Heaths focus more on the environment's effect and how this can be used for positive ends.

The overlaps for success are: a strong narrative leading to a clear endpoint; the need to make change seem possible through 'inch pebbles' (mini-milestones); the benefits of the many driving change rather than opposing or at least doing nothing; and finally the need to create habits.

Using the example of St Anywhere Hospital, the benefits of these approaches can be seen. For the cataract patient pathway at St Anywhere Hospital, efficiency, productivity, safety and satisfaction could be improved by creating a simpler pathway based around the one-stop shop concept and ultimately run by non-doctors. The evidence and a toolkit for change in this area is available from the National Institute for Improvement and Innovation (NHSI).

TABLE 11.1 Applying lessons from Kotter and Heath to St Anywhere ophthalmology service

Kotter	Heath	St Anywhere
	Follow the bright spots (identify positive change stories)	Listen to the stories from the NHSI
Communicate the vision	Script the change	Lay out the steps:
		Streamline pre-op care assessments
		Increase throughput through theatre
		Outsource post-op care to the community

Kotter	Heath	St Anywhere
Elucidate a clear vision	Point to the destination	One-stop shops and reduced visits to hospital
Create a sense of urgency	Find the feeling (inspire through positive emotion)	Bring patient who has experienced one-stop shop to monthly meeting Map the current pathway
Create short-term wins	Shrink the change (create 'inch pebbles')	Delineate the steps in bite-size pieces, e.g. start with nurses doing biometry for every patient
Create coalition	Grow your people (develop a momentum based on identity)	Reward the nurses who take on more with increased training opportunities Work with patient groups to promote the change locally
	Tweak the environment	Re-orientate the workflow
Consolidate improvements Institutionalise new approaches	Build habits	Create cataract clinics so that the learning processes can happen quickly
Empowering others to act	Rally the herd (effects can spread)	Start with one consultant and spread

Looking at Table 11.1, it is possible to see how to proceed. First, identifying change that works both from materials available from the NHS Institute for Innovation and Improvement; then to elucidate and express the goal: creating a one-stop shop and streamlined care pathway for cataracts; in addition, creating a real-time focus by communicating to the local GPs that this is St Anywhere's vision. In addition, the order of events becomes important: first, streamline pre-operative care, so that visits include measurements for surgery; pre-assessment by anaesthetics and consent all happen in one short visit rather than multiple seemingly unending visits.

Moving on to the emotional: to create the emotional commitment to change, bringing patients to the monthly unit meeting who have experienced this sort of arrangement elsewhere, who can talk with passion about why it matters, would be a positive enforcer and motivator. Alternatively, to create a burning platform the current pathway could be drawn on a wall and the implications in the new Payment by Results (PbR) tariff explored. The 2010–11 tariff creates a bundled payment for cataract, which is less than the current total for the pathway as carried out by St Anywhere, but more than the one-stop pathways could be charged at. *See* Chapter 9 for more explanation of PbR. This is followed by improvements to surgical productivity, via training of a few early adopter community optometrists in post-operative care in the community. The inch pebbles might commence with small wins like empowering the nurses to take over new functions such as biometry. Similarly, rewarding those nurses who do so with further training, and involving patients groups to push the change, helps to build the coalition.

Altering the physical layout such that the rooms are close enough together helps, as does having a post-box system so that when patients are finished with one bit of their visit, they can display readiness for the next by posting their card through the relevant door (thereby gaining attention without distracting the work of a clinician). The sheer volume of cataracts, or other procedure, means that patterns can be created, especially if all those with potential cataracts are streamed and booked into a few concentrated cataract-specific clinics. Finally, if the focus is on one consultant and then clinical curiosity and competition is used to spread the change, the whole unit might soon have 'switched'.

None of the above will happen by accident. Someone has to will it, to make the change happen. To use the terminology of the best known behavioural economics book, *Nudge*, someone has to be the choice architect. This is the person who assesses and manipulates the environment, using their knowledge of behavioural traits for the benefit of the programme. In *Nudge*, Thaler and Sunstein brilliantly address how through understanding behavioural economics, change particularly at the policy level can be gently created rather than being regimented through laws or left to arise of its own in a libertarian world. Instead, they advocate liberal paternalism. This means guiding choices to the best end point (as determined by those with detailed knowledge). Thaler and Sunstein sum up their approach to NUDGE people as: iNcentivise, Understand mappings (the systems to change), use Defaults, Give feedback, Expect error and Structure complex choices. (*See* Table 11.2 for examples that aid definitions.)

For St Anywhere and their programme to improve DNA rates this might look like Table 11.2.

TABLE 11.2 NUDGES for St Anywhere

iNcentivise	Create a monthly award for the greatest improvement in DNA rates
Understand mappings	Create a call centre that calls patients a week before their next appointment and asks them to choose an appointment in the following week
use Defaults	In the above system the default is thus an expectation that the patient will forget to attend
Give feedback	Publish monthly DNA rates publicly
Expect errors	Understand that some patient groups are more likely to DNA and build a 'handicap system' to acknowledge this
Structure complex choices	Take the system of follow up appointments out of the hands of busy receptionists into an offsite, calm 24/7 call centre with multiple languages

This chapter has used a few examples from the burgeoning literature about how to make change occur. To date, very little has been consciously or consistently applied to healthcare. Concepts of behavioural economics are likely to become more central to themes of change in the NHS. Major political parties are enthused by the concepts that have been applied to other policy areas. (Thaler, author of *Nudge*, is one of David Cameron's advisors, and the book *Connected*, which looks at the influence of individuals within their networks, is widely talked about within Conservative circles.)

MINDSPACE is a report published by the Institute for Government (2010). It is effectively *Nudge* for policy creation. It provides a framework to apply the concepts of behavioural economics when developing new policies. Table 11.3 identifies the key points brought out by the report.

TABLE 11.3 MINDSPACE

Concept	Definition
Messenger	We are heavily influenced by who communicates information
Incentives	Our responses to incentives are shaped by predictable mental shortcuts, such as strongly avoiding losses
Norms	We are strongly influenced by what others do
Defaults	We 'go with the flow' of pre-set options
Salience	Our attention is drawn to what is novel and seems relevant to us
Priming	Our acts are often influenced by sub-conscious cues
Affect	Our emotional associations can powerfully shape our actions
Commitments	We seek to be consistent with our public promises, and reciprocate acts
Ego	We act in ways that make us feel better about ourselves

SUMMARY

This chapter has hopefully excited the reader about change and provided a range of frameworks to aid change, alongside examples from St Anywhere Hospital of how this might work in practice. The application of the principles of behavioural economics to healthcare is at an early stage in its development. This chapter has demonstrated that there is much potential for future research in this field.

The following chapter explores the world of quality improvement, which walks hand-in-hand with concepts of change management.

FURTHER READING

Ariely D (2009). *Predictably Irrational*. Revised ed. London: HarperCollins Publishers.

Berry LL, Seltman KD (2008). *Management Lessons from Mayo Clinic*. New York: McGraw Hill.

Brafman O, Brafman R (2008). *Sway*. New York: DoubleDay.

Christakis N, Fowler J (2010). *Connected: the amazing power of social networks and how they shape our lives*. New York: HarperPress.

Dolan A, Hallsworth M, Halpern D, *et al*. (2010). *MINDSPACE*. London: The Cabinet Office. Available at: www.civilservice.gov.uk/news/2010/march/mindspace.aspx (accessed 20 April 2010).

Earls M (2009). *Herd: how to change mass behaviour by harnessing our true behaviour*. Revised ed. Chichester: John Wiley & Sons, Ltd.

Heath D, Heath C (2010). *Switch: how to change things when change is hard*. London: Random House Business Books.

Kotter J (1995). Leading change: why transformation efforts fail. *Harvard Business Review*; 1–10.

Lehrer J (2009). *The Decisive Moment: how the brain makes up its mind.* Edinburgh: Canongate Books Ltd.

Thaler RH, Cass R (2009). *Nudge: improving decisions about health, wealth and happiness.* Revised ed. London: Penguin Group.

CHAPTER 12

Quality streets

Some is not a number. Soon is not a time.

Don Berwick, Institute for Healthcare Improvement

INTRODUCTION

Lord Darzi's Next Stage Review (DH, 2008) shone a spotlight on quality as the organising principle of the NHS. This chapter reviews the origins of quality improvement from the manufacturing industry and considers how these approaches have been implemented into healthcare, in particular in the NHS to date. The second half of this chapter looks at the practical application of quality improvement methodology to healthcare, learning from the inspirational Institute for Healthcare Improvement (IHI), USA.

QUALITY

In industry, ensuring quality saves organisations. In healthcare, ensuring quality saves lives. Chapter 3 has summarised the Institute of Medicine's definition of quality in healthcare across six dimensions (safe, effective, patient-centred, timely, efficient and equitable).

The term 'quality improvement' (QI) is frequently misunderstood in healthcare. Lack of knowledge and experience about quality improvement is one of the key barriers to successful implementation in the NHS.

Quality improvement is defined as a complex social intervention involving inter-related processes such as training, teamwork, data feedback and support. Hockey and Marshall (2009) advocate educational solutions as the key to this in both undergraduate and postgraduate training programmes. Clinicians in the US are more familiar with applying quality improvement methods to their clinical working environments than doctors in the UK. There are moves to change this. For example, the London Deanery and the Royal College of Physicians are currently discussing making 'quality improvement projects' mandatory for all trainees during their training, instead of audit projects. Boxes 12.1 and 12.2 give examples of Foundation Year 1 doctors' quality improvement projects, carried out in teams, at Salisbury NHS Foundation Trust (reproduced with permission from Professor Peter Wilcock, Director of Service Improvement). Salisbury NHS Foundation Trust has been engaging junior doctors in quality improvement methodology to inform cycles of change since 2005, known as HImP (Interprofessional Healthcare Improvement Programme for Junior Staff). The junior doctors identify target areas for improvement, with guidance. This enables the projects to be both important to the doctors and to leave a legacy of value to the Trust. The boxes illustrate the ongoing nature of quality improvement.

Experience from the US suggests that doing many small-scale projects may lead to difficulty in achieving wide-scale system change. Therefore, in an environment where many quality improvement projects are being simultaneously undertaken, there is a need to align projects to an overall strategic vision to achieve maximum results, for example, reducing suicide rates or hospital-acquired infection rates to zero. As junior doctors are not in positions of power, they may be best placed to undertake QI as team members.

BOX 12.1 Improving the speed and reliability of internal consultant-to-consultant referrals, Salisbury NHS Foundation Trust

The current system involved one team writing an A6 pink slip containing clinical details of the patient and reason for referral, delivering this pink slip to the relevant secretary who would pass the slip to the team, culminating in the specialist team reviewing the patient and taking over their care if appropriate. The current system was considered very time consuming and unreliable. Hence this was identified as an area for quality improvement.

The process of the current system was mapped using a process map, highlighting each stage involved. The group of trainees tracked a variety of slips from various specialties and found that referral to review times varied from 2 hours to 10 days. The goal of the project was to standardise these times.

A box system was trialled in the gastroenterology department, where teams requesting referral could deposit a slip on the ward, rather than taking it to the secretaries. This trial resulted in a reduction of referral to review time to a maximum of three days. This was well received by junior doctors, as assessed by questionnaire.

The second change involved the redesign of the pink slip itself. This was outdated and contained little clinical information. In conjunction with other members of the development team, the trainees designed a new slip containing more relevant clinical information, a box specifying whether the referring team wished the review team to simply review or take over their care, a box specifying expected date of discharge if known, and made sticky backed to enable consultants to stick the slip in the notes as a record of referral and consultation.

BOX 12.2 Improving communication with medical staff on call, Salisbury NHS Foundation Trust

The aim of this project was to improve the system for contacting the on-call junior doctors for medicine and surgery. The on-call junior doctors were receiving a very high number of non-urgent bleeps over the course of their shift. This was reducing the amount of time they were able to spend seeing patients and completing their work. Data was collected over several weekends prior to making a change. On average, the Foundation Year 1 (F1) doctor on-call for medicine was spending more than 90 minutes answering their bleep. Nursing staff were finding it time consuming having to contact switchboard to find out the on-call bleep number for the medical F1, as there was no baton bleep, so the number constantly changed depending who was on call. A process map and a fish bone analysis were carried out to establish where changes could be made to improve the system.

A baton bleep was introduced for the medical F1 on ward cover. A survey revealed very positive feedback. The biggest difference was in the amount of time nursing staff spent finding out the number they needed to bleep. In addition, switchboard operators also found it an improvement, as they did not have to remember a new number every time a different person was on call.

The second problem identified as a group of trainees was the large number of non-urgent bleeps that the F1 on ward cover received. This was disruptive and often meant that tasks took much longer than they needed to. The group met with the IT (Information Technology) department to discuss potential solutions. In conjunction with the IT department, an electronic task list was created using the consultant list system. This enabled nurses to enter jobs on to the F1's list so that the F1 could then look at the list when convenient, and prioritise the jobs accordingly. Urgent jobs would still be bleeped through as previously. (This system is currently being piloted on two wards in Salisbury Hospital.)

HISTORY OF QUALITY IMPROVEMENT

Industrial approaches to quality improvement were developed in the manufacturing industry before the Second World War. The mass production required during the Second World War brought these individuals together and converged their approaches. Over the last 50 years, the quality movement in manufacturing has developed from the tools and techniques of individual specialists to become company-wide approaches. In industry, the quality movement occurred in two waves: first, from 1945 onwards; and second as a relaunch in the 1980s.

The different approaches to quality improvement can be used individually or, as is more likely in healthcare, in combination. They are based on similar common principles and represent a convergence of approaches rather than being uniquely different. The common themes are: customer is central to everything; work processes should be categorised, redesigned if necessary, and understood as part of a wider system; measure components of the process and understand the importance of variation in these measures; recognise and value the expertise in people working on the front line.

Juran suggested that customer satisfaction should be the chief operating goal. Recent initiatives in the NHS have moved towards gaining feedback from the patient on their experience as a customer, through Patient Reported Outcome Measures (PROMs). At present, these are linked to a small amount of NHS Trusts' incomes. The NHS is currently faced with the conundrum of reducing costs while endeavouring to improve quality. The evidence that this is possible is unconvincing.

The Total Quality Movement (TQM) emerged from post-war Japan. At this time, Japanese plants were observed to be twice as good as their Western counterparts. TQM is defined as a 'management approach for an organisation, centred on quality, based on the participation of all its members and aiming at long-term success through customer satisfaction, and benefits to all members of the organisation and to society' (International Organization for Standardization, 1994).

In Japan, TQM comprises four steps:

> ➤ Kaizen – 'Continuous Process Improvement' to make processes visible, repeatable and measurable.
> ➤ Atarimae Hinshitsu – the idea that 'things will work as they are supposed to'.
> ➤ Kansei – examining the way the user applies the product leads to improvement in the product itself.
> ➤ Miryokuteki Hinshitsu – the idea that 'things should have an aesthetic quality'.

The use of TQM in healthcare increased in the 1990s, although it has had little impact on the work of medical staff. There is limited evidence about its effectiveness in healthcare and whether it is better or worse than any other quality improvement approaches.

Plan-do-study-act (PDSA) cycles are small tests of change used as part of a continuous improvement approach (Deming). The practitioner *plans* a test of change, then carries out the change (*do*), *studies* the results and then *acts* on them in the next cycle of change. PDSA has been widely used in healthcare (Boxes 12.1 and 12.2), championed by leading figures such as Don Berwick, IHI. PDSA is sometimes used as part of Lean and in Six Sigma. The impact has been shown to rely on the participants, their host organisation and the style and method of implementation. There is no evidence to suggest that PDSA is more cost-effective than any other approach to improve quality in healthcare, and the longer-term impact has not been evaluated.

Statistical process control (SPC) has been widely promoted as a key tool in TQM, Six Sigma, Theory of Constraints and the PDSA cycle. Shewhart initially identified the difference between 'natural' variation in measures of a process (common cause) and 'special' variation that can be controlled. Processes showing only common cause variation are said to be in statistical control. The central tool is a control chart that adds process variation bounds as upper and lower control limits (typically ±2 or 2 standard deviations) to a run chart of time.

SPC has a wide application in healthcare to report performance data at board level and to provide guidance for health professionals on treatment effectiveness. The awareness of SPC in the UK was raised following its application to data about mortality in the Shipman case and the Bristol inquiry. Systematic review has shown that SPC improves communication between clinicians, managers and patients. It does this by providing a shared language to describe and quantify variation, to identify areas for potential improvement and to assess the impact of change interventions. There is no evidence that it reduces the cost of healthcare. The limitations of SPC are the complexity of data sets in terms of aggregations of different types of patients, and the implications of the data set being very large or very small. Whilst SPC can be effective in healthcare, it requires greater skills and training than other approaches and is dependent on good quality data, which is often lacking, largely due to coding error and a lack of engagement of frontline clinicians with aggregate data sets.

Six Sigma was developed by Motorola in the 1980s and originates from Shewhart and Deming's earlier work, described above. Six Sigma enabled Motorola to express its quality goal as 3.4 defects per million opportunities (DPMO), where a defect opportunity is a process output that fails to meet the customer's critical requirements. Errors in healthcare are not measured in this way, which makes it difficult to compare rates. Six Sigma is a philosophy of identifying customer needs and then establishing the root causes of variation in meeting these needs. There is a certification structure for levels of competence in applying the approach (master black, black and green 'belts'). There are structured methodologies: *define, measure, analyse, improve* and *control* (DMAIC). There are a variety of tools for improvement, including process mapping and SPC. Six Sigma aims to eliminate defects and reduce variation in a process to improve output and outcomes from the system. Six Sigma has been widely applied to healthcare over the last decade. From the literature, its effectiveness is mainly descriptive and lacks systematic evaluation.

There are five principles of Lean: identify customer value, manage the value stream, 'flow' production, pull work through the process and pursue perfection by reducing all forms of waste in the system. This is summarised in the 'Toyota Production System' (TPS) as the 'Toyota Way: problem-solving, people and partners, process and philosophy'. Lean is often integrated with other approaches such as Six Sigma to become Lean Six Sigma.

Value Stream Mapping (VSM) analyses the flow of resources to categorise waste into seven categories, shown in table 12.1 with healthcare examples.

TABLE 12.1 Value stream mapping

Lean waste category	Healthcare examples
Correction (defects)	Adverse drug reactions
	Readmission because of inappropriate discharge
	Repeat tests because of incorrect information
Waiting	Waiting for doctors to discharge patients
	Waiting for test results
Transportation	Central equipment stores rather than ward-based stores
Over processing	Asking patients for the same information several times
Inventory	Waiting lists
	Excess stock in stockrooms
Motion	Unnecessary staff movements to obtain information or supplies
Overproduction	Requesting unnecessary tests
	Keeping beds free 'just in case'

5S (or CANDO – Clean up, Arrange, Neatness, Discipline, Ongoing improvement) is the 'basic housekeeping discipline for Lean, quality and safety':

➤ **Sort** – classify equipment and supplies by frequency of use, remove what is not used.
➤ **Simplify/straighten/set in order** – allocate a place for equipment and supplies and standardise locations.
➤ **Shine/scrub** – clean and check.

➤ **Standardise/Stabilise** – adopt standard work and standards for 5S.
➤ **Sustain/Self Discipline** – ongoing 5S, housekeeping audits.

Rapid Improvement Events (RIE) are seen as 'the engine for implementing the changes (physical and cultural) that a Lean approach requires'. These are four- or five-day events aimed at analysing current processes and identifying changes needed. There are many 'how to' guides to implement Lean into NHS. However, there is currently no robust evidence base to support this application into a service industry such as healthcare.

APPLICATION FOR HEALTHCARE

In England, the Care Quality Commission (CQC) is the independent regulator for health and social care. Although the aim of CQC is to ensure better care for everyone, Deming would call this 'reliance on inspection to improve'. W Edward Deming was one of the 'quality gurus' who developed a management philosophy to improve quality in industry in the early 1950s. His approach has been influential in improving quality in both the manufacturing industry and in applying this model to healthcare.

The Institute for Healthcare Improvement (IHI), USA, has pioneered the application of quality improvement methods from industry into healthcare. IHI uses Deming's 'system of profound knowledge' in four interrelated parts: appreciation for a system, understanding variation, building knowledge and the human side of change (discussed in Chapter 12). The Model for Improvement, used by IHI to apply improvement theory to healthcare, consists of three key questions:
➤ What are we trying to accomplish?
➤ How will we know that a change is an improvement?
➤ What change can we make that will result in an improvement?

Don Berwick, from IHI, has written the following about The Model for Improvement:

> This model is not magic, but it is probably the most useful single framework I have encountered in twenty years of my own work in quality improvement. It can guide teams, support reflection, and provide an outline for oversight and review; it is thoroughly portable, applying usefully in myriad contexts.

The approach for healthcare is that improving quality is pragmatic as well as intellectual. There is great emphasis placed on doing the improvement work, as opposed to long periods of time spent learning about it. The above three questions are a quick and memorable formula. However, do not be fooled into thinking that system improvement is simple. All improvement requires change but not all change leads to improvement. Chapter 12 explores management of change. Change is difficult and requires a sustainable, team-based approach.

Changing a tyre or changing a light bulb because they have worn out are reactions to problems rather than changes for improvement. Change is often resisted to defend the status quo. This is the approach of 'If it ain't broke, don't fix it'. It is true that attempting change may make things worse. To prevent this, learning is linked to testing through the PDSA cycle described previously. This aims to lead to effective redesign. However, the following ingredients are required for success:

➤ Strong leadership and people management (Chapter 7).
➤ Better ideas with examples that have been successfully implemented.
➤ Clear plan to include lines of communication, measurement and work.

For quality improvement to be successful, it is not possible to jump straight from idea to implementation. The process must involve testing and constant referral to the three questions about what is trying to be accomplished and how it will be measured throughout the process.

The testing phase will include the who, where, when, what and how. Following each test, the process should be adapted and repeated as a cycle. The Shewhart charts described above offer a mechanism to capture data. These can help to identify whether a change in the data is because something has changed or because it is random.

Some of the key challenges to overcome when thinking about quality improvement are listed below:

➤ Time to meet the objective. For doctors, this means balancing time spent on quality improvement of the service versus time spent on service delivery.
➤ Thinking of a change that will lead to improvement. Creative thinking is best done in teams.
➤ Motivating participation. Getting people to participate in yet another activity on top of their existing workload is an undeniable challenge. A competition and/or awards may be a useful carrot to dangle.
➤ Recognise when change leads to improvement. Kotter (Chapter 11) encourages celebrating small successes to facilitate a movement for change.
➤ The 'improvement evaporation effect' (lack sustainability).

Monovoxoplegia is 'paralysis by one loud voice'. This is a common phenomenon in doctors' meetings and board meetings. The majority may sit silent, as bystanders, while one individual speaks up against a proposed change. Showing courage is the best antidote to monovoxoplegia. The best thing about courage is that it is infectious.

To spread a change means adopting it by more than one team, in more than one ward, in more than one hospital, in more than one Strategic Health Authority. Investing in building capability throughout an organisation is essential to sustaining improvement, as in Salisbury Hospital with their leading approach to engaging junior doctors in quality improvement. Boxes 12.1 and 12.2 are examples of the power of timely data collection and communication, to proving how the change has enhanced the quality of care as defined earlier, through for example, improving patient safety, or reducing waiting time for patients. There is considerable evidence of high failure rates in projects sustaining their efforts (as much as 70%).

> Improvement efforts will only succeed if the same effort is put into their sustainability as their launch.
>
> (Health Service Management Centre, 2002)

Following on from the chapter on change management, to 'nudge' people most effectively into making a change, first, communicate the problem and second, introduce the new idea using data to show how the situation has improved. Rogers' adoption curve for innovation, in the following chapter, suggests focusing initially on the early adopters to build the evidence for success and then disseminating more widely.

SUMMARY

This chapter has provided an overview of quality improvement methodology and reviewed how this has been applied to healthcare. Successful improvement depends on teams working together interprofessionally to design improvements to the care they provide to their patients. A key legacy of such projects is the improved working relationships they leave behind, which may be more enduring than the redesigned processes themselves. The locus of control of the change is crucial, i.e. people may not resist change so much as resist being changed. Leadership, discussed in Chapter 7, is key to the sustained success of quality improvement efforts.

At present, the experience of transferring quality improvement techniques into the NHS has not reached widespread success. Chapter 12 has explained that success or failure depends as much on how the change is managed as the new technique or change itself. As opposed to the NHS copying and pasting the American IHI blueprint approach to quality improvement, we propose there is great potential for international healthcare systems to share learning for the gain of all.

FURTHER READING

Bendell T (1992). *The Quality Gurus*. London: Department of Trade and Industry.

Crump B, Adil M (2009). Can quality and productivity be improved in a financially poorer NHS? *BMJ*; **339**: b4638.

Department of Health (2008). *Next Stage Review*. London: Department of Health.

Hockey PM, Marshall MN (2009). Doctors and quality improvement. *Journal of Royal Society of Medicine*; **102**: 173–6.

Institute of Medicine (2001). *Crossing the Quality Chasm: a new health system for the 21st century*. Washington, DC: National Academy Press.

Langley GJ, Moen R, Nolan KM, *et al.* (2009). *The Improvement Guide: a practical approach to enhancing organizational performance*. San Francisco, CA: Jossey Bass.

Powell AE, Rushmer RK, Davies HTO (2009). A systematic narrative review of quality improvement models in health care. *NHS Quality Improvement Scotland*. The Universities of Dundee and St Andrews.

Reinertsen JL, Bisognano M, Pugh MD (2008). *Seven Leadership Leverage Points for Organization-level Improvement in Health Care*. 2nd ed. Cambridge, MA: Institute for Healthcare Improvement.

Rogers EM (1962). *Diffusion of Innovations*. Glencoe: Free Press.

CHAPTER 13

Doctorpreneur

It sounded an excellent plan, no doubt, and very neatly and simply arranged.

The only difficulty was, she had not the smallest idea how to set about it.

Lewis Carroll, Alice in Alice in Wonderland

INTRODUCTION

en•tre•pre•neur – noun entrepreneur, translated from its French roots, means 'one who undertakes'. The term entrepreneur refers to anyone who undertakes the organisation and management of an enterprise involving independence and risk as well as the opportunity for profit.

Despite the current financial climate of caution, there is a strong and defiant entrepreneurial aspiration palpable amongst 'Generation Y'. Twenty-four per cent of young Britons say their dream job is to run their own business (YouGov, 2010). This survey (of over 2000 people) identified the key barriers to people achieving their ambitions as concerns about having the right contacts or experience. Although commercial experience and training may be a potential barrier to doctors running their own business, a lack of contacts certainly isn't. The current training model for doctors, of rotating placements every 4–6 months, rapidly enables trainees to make many links across different networks.

Despite its current popularity, entrepreneurship is a relatively new entry to the MBA syllabus. As yet, it remains notably absent from medical undergraduate and postgraduate training.

Many people argue that entrepreneurship cannot be taught. The only way to learn it is to do it. Subsequently, this is the way many business schools teach entrepreneurship, by supporting groups to come up with an innovative idea and guiding them through all of the steps to take the product to market. Many people who do an MBA are already entrepreneurs. Others do an MBA to become more commercially savvy, to either grow their existing business or to leave their current employment to set up their own company. This chapter provides practical advice about how to set up a business, including real-life case studies of doctors who have become entrepreneurs: what we term, doctorpreneurs. To set the inspirational scene, Box 13.1 shares the story of one successful doctorpreneur who combined his medical experience with his pre-existing networks to build a successful company.

DOCTORPRENEURS

Medics with MBAs are in an ideal position to become healthcare entrepreneurs, a career option discussed further in Chapter 16. As well as the explicit subject matter learnt on an MBA, one of the implicit skills acquired from an MBA is the confidence to 'have a go'. This is crucial to being an entrepreneur.

Clinicians' proximity to patients and knowledge of disease makes them ideally placed to be innovators of healthcare services. The incentive to act in an entrepreneurial fashion goes beyond financial gain. The critical benefit of creating a culture in healthcare where entrepreneurship is encouraged is direct and indirect improvement of patient care.

Richard Branson is passionate that inspiring people to think like entrepreneurs by giving them more responsibility will improve their performance. Professor Jenny Simpson shares her views on the capability of junior clinicians to identify new market niches and act on them in Box 13.2.

However attractive and fun setting up and running a business alongside being a clinician sounds, the reality is that it is beset with challenges. The majority of new businesses fail and so having a thick skin is essential for survival.

The doctorpreneurism ability displayed in Box 13.1 is an example of the broader ability of clinicians, to innovate to find solutions to problems. We have discovered many examples of innovations by medics, often early on in their training, but seldom are these immense efforts recognised.

Box 13.1 is also an example of the opportunities for international entrepreneurism. Unlike working in the NHS, doing an MBA encourages students to think in terms of a global market. There are broadly four main categories in which healthcare can be traded: first, exporting or importing health services via electronic means; second, exporting health services by importing patients; third, exporting or importing foreign direct investment (FDI); and fourth, by exporting or importing healthcare professionals.

The trend for medical tourism is a rapidly innovating and growing field. India has a 15–20% year-on-year growth in healthcare tourism. Over 1.2 million health tourists visited Thailand in 2005. Singapore aims to treat 1 million healthcare tourists with revenue of $3 billion by 2012. In Europe, the medical tourist market is estimated to be €1 billion per year.

New opportunities for doctorpreneurs in international healthcare are not just in medical tourism. Lord Nigel Crisp, former Chief Executive and Permanent Secretary for the NHS, was asked by then Prime Minister Tony Blair to explore how the expertise of the NHS could be used, not for medical tourism, but to improve health in developing countries. Nigel Crisp's findings were that rich countries, such as the UK, could learn a great deal about health and health services from poorer ones, and that the key to improving health would be to combine insights from both rich and poor countries. Nigel Crisp identified many examples of healthcare professionals innovating and creating new solutions to their problems in poor countries simply because they had to: 'Although resource-poor, the medical staff were far from knowledge-poor'. Many of these innovations have applicability for healthcare in the rich West.

BOX 13.1 Doctorpreneurism in action

Medics often have, for one reason or another, a fantastic knack of seeing opportunities, but a paralleled inability to capitalise.

Having been a victim of this myself over many years, I found the solution: partnership. My story involves countless missed communications following outpatient sessions, where my dictated letters sat untyped and fallow in the secretary's dungeons, lost amidst bundles of disorganised files.

I'd seen how the Americans did it, through outsourcing dictation to India. This facilitated the cheap and quick turnaround of important letters, and led to better, more co-ordinated and safer patient care. So how could I do it in the UK, not only to help patients, but also to make a buck?

I went to my friend, a management consultant, and told him of the idea. Immediately, his training kicked in and he started analysing things in ways I poorly understood – opportunity cost, risk analysis, time to market, competitor propositions – and luckily decided within 30 minutes that it was a jolly good idea.

So we set about drawing up a business plan (not for investment, but to give us clear direction), and put a few thousand pounds each into it. Then we sorted out our diaries to make sure we made the time to make this work.

So why did it work? Well I knew the market, he knew business process. I had the contacts, he had the sales experience. I had the customer insight, he had the delivery programme.

Between us, we were working as a single unit. I knew the environment, and told him about the issues and opportunities in plain English. He then translated these into business speak (educating me along the way), and once I found myself analysing RFP (request for proposal) responses from potential suppliers according to a criteria matrix, I knew this was going to work.

Within one year, we had sold a large number of contracts, often through places I'd worked as a clinician previously, and where I knew there were issues. I knew who to approach, and how to approach them, and this was key.

Spurred on by more contracts, we were bought out for a significant sum and the experience not only made me money but also taught me the ropes of business. The lesson I will always take with me is that getting the right people on the right tasks and working cohesively is a very probable path to success.

BOX 13.2 Rocking the boat

Professor Jenny Simpson, Chief Executive of BAMM
(British Association of Medical Managers)

Young doctors are bright, often highly creative, highly energised people. It is hardly surprising that some of them have very highly developed entrepreneurial skills. What is more surprising is that the establishment does not harness young bright brains and use them to their full potential. As any other industry would do.

Rather, the system tends to somewhat distain new ideas from anywhere other than the traditional academic world of scientific breakthrough, double blind trails and learned papers.

(continued)

Instead of encouraging innovative thinking in junior doctors, the tradition has been – apart from in a small number of forward-thinking organisations – to ignore it. One might be forgiven for thinking that the system secretly hopes that it will soon exhaust and drain the energy away from anything that might disrupt it.

What if a pair of fresh bright eyes, close to patients and the clinical frontline, happens to spot a new way of doing things that improves the process, the way patients feel or maybe a radical way of communicating key information to clinicians who work at strange times of the day and night? What if those fresh eyes see ways through problems that others, with their eyes tired from being so close and their minds, brainwashed and stuck in a groove of 'this is how it is and always will be' – have tried for years to solve? What if those new ideas cause discomfort?

Huge, complex, publicly funded organisations are not on the whole given to welcoming entrepreneurial thinking. Indeed, an indicator of how well the would-be entrepreneur is doing can be measured in terms of the number of times per day they are told to '*not rock the boat, doctor*' . . . Yet, the complexity of running healthcare, free for all at the point of delivery is unlikely to become miraculously easy over the next few years of financial constraint. And it may just be that the NHS can no longer afford to ignore the innovative ideas of its junior doctors.

INNOVATION

> Innovation is no longer one of those 'nice things to do' if we have a bit of time to spare. It's business critical and all of us in the NHS need to be looking for new, improved ways of using our resources to deliver the best services, every day.
>
> *David Nicholson CBE, Chief Executive NHS*

Being an entrepreneur demands innovation. Not just for products and technology but also for services. Innovation in services is relatively under-researched. However, service innovation is increasingly overdue for healthcare. Over the last 20 years, the number of hospital beds in the NHS has reduced from 270 000 to 160 000. This has only been possible due to innovation in a combination of products, technology and services. Innovation can be categorised in a number of ways, depending on its features and uses. Examples of categories of innovation are given below.

One example of product innovation in healthcare is gall bladder removal. This can now take place through keyhole surgery, requiring only one day in hospital, rather than invasive surgery, which used to require seven.

Process innovation in healthcare is required to identify new solutions for managing long-term conditions. One example of this is a telephone-based care system in Birmingham, where people with chronic conditions can directly contact nurses to discuss their disease or medication. This scheme has halved hospital attendance amongst those who use it. Another process innovation is the idea of a 'virtual ward', where people identified as being at risk of an emergency hospital admission are being admitted instead to a 'virtual ward'. They can then be looked after by a team of health professionals in the community in their own home. Dr Geraint Lewis, a public health doctor, developed this idea that identifies those 'at risk' using a computerised predictive tool, building on his experience working in hospital care. This analyses individual patient data, including information about hospital, outpatient and accident and emergency admissions and attendances as well as information about the frequency of using GP services. Once admitted to the virtual ward, patients are looked after at different levels of intensity and reviewed by a multi-agency team on a daily basis. The final example of process innovation comes from the Virginia Mason Medical Centre, Seattle, USA. Here, medical teams have learnt from the 'drive-through' success of fast-food restaurants and offer 'drive-through' influenza vaccinations.

Radical innovation is a concept that fundamentally changes the way things are done and frequently leads to a new industry. James Watson and Francis Crick's unravelling the structure of DNA in 1953, led to the human genome project, completed in 2003, which has revolutionised the science of genetics. Radical innovation is sometimes called 'disruptive technology' and is often competence-destroying. This means it may make previous skills obsolete as it requires new knowledge, expertise and assets. Incremental innovation is about making incremental improvements to an existing technology. This might be the identification of another gene. Incremental innovations tend to be competence-enhancing. This means they build on existing knowledge and expertise rather than requiring new knowledge and expertise.

Architectural innovation is when the components of a product or process change. In healthcare, one example is changing from hypodermic injections to pills. Component innovation occurs when changes between the components (architecture) and between the product and the user change. One healthcare example of component innovation is the transfer of information between individuals. This has evolved from using floppy discs or CDs to transferring content or patient information via online networks and downloads. This has led to rapid improvements globally in the rate of dissemination of evidence-based medicine and the development of the

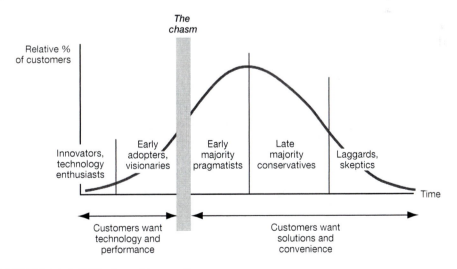

FIGURE 13.1 Diffusion of innovation

Source: Moore G (1998). *Crossing the Chasm: marketing and selling technology products to mainstream customers*. Oxford: Capstone.

electronic patient record (EPR). Component innovations are frequently incremental.

At present, healthcare delivery remains largely orientated around one-to-one face-to-face meetings between patients and doctors. However, much of this could be carried out over the internet. One example of this is computerised cognitive behavioural therapy, which has broadened access to psychological therapies. At Kaiser Permanente, USA, patients are able to email questions and receive a response from a specialist within 72 hours. Patients are also encouraged to access their laboratory results and vaccination history, and order prescriptions as well as appointments online.

The adoption of innovation can be visualised as a normal distribution curve. Figure 13.1 illustrates Rogers' (1962) basic segmentation of adopters of innovation. The different categories of adopters vary according to resources, affinity for risk, knowledge, socio-economic status, need and interest in the product. Moore's (1991) chasm is highlighted. The chasm is a crucial opportunity for entrepreneurs. The transition from early adopters to an early majority frequently requires a leap in competencies and a different product concept, either in training or pricing or service support. The model of diffusion in Figure 13.1 also applies to the diffusion of quality improvement approaches, discussed in the preceding chapter.

Peter Jones, successful entrepreneur of *Dragons' Den* fame, made his fortune with Phones International Group – not by making or changing mobile phones but by being the 'middle man' that could 'cross the chasm' and sell mobile phones to the majority. This is an example of process innovation.

LEGAL ARCHITECTURE

Once the innovation is realised, there is a mind-boggling array of bureaucracy attached to taking the new idea to market. Lord Sugar, with more than 40 years experience in starting and growing businesses, likens the administrative obstacles involved to the Grand National. In true *Apprentice* style, his advice is to just, 'Get on with it'. With that in mind, below is an overview of initial steps designed to help in setting up your own company.

1. Incorporating a company

The Companies Act (2006) contains the necessary requirements for company registration. Companies House is an Executive Agency of the Department for Business, Innovation and Skills (BIS) and registers companies. Every year, more than 300 000 new companies are registered and there are over 2 million limited companies in Great Britain. In addition to incorporating limited companies, Companies House also dissolves them, stores company information and makes it available to the public.

To incorporate a limited company, details of the directors and share capital need to be submitted to Companies House as well as the Memorandum of Association and the Articles of Association. Proformas of these documents are easily accessible online.

2. Set up a bank account

To facilitate an end-of-year tax return as well as gaining access to a range of other services, it is advisable to have a separate business bank account for your company rather than use your personal bank account. Most high-street banks will offer free 'Business Banking' services for the first two years. In addition to traditional banking services, these accounts frequently include access to online courses, invoice systems and direct access to a personal bank manager. There may also be advantageous bank loans available to help start up your company, if required. Other sources of funding to consider include approaching business angels, venture capital, a strategic partner or accessing subsidies and awards.

3. Register for VAT

Value Added Tax (VAT) is a tax on most business transactions in the UK. VAT is not payable until your turnover has reached £68 000. Once you have reached this threshold, you have 30 days to register online before breaching. Once registered for VAT it is possible to both charge VAT on the goods and services you provide and also reclaim VAT on anything you purchase for your business.

4. Business insurance

Even if you don't have premises initially, business insurance is important. Your bank or membership organisations, such as the Institute of Directors, may be able to offer preferential rates for insurance. As with all insurance policies, it is worth shopping around for competitive rates. Even if you are not in office premises, there may be a need for public liability, employee liability, indemnity insurance and insurance for specific items such as office equipment and computers.

5. Set up a website

Undoubtedly getting online as soon as possible is good for your business. There are many free or cheaply available packages which allow you to rapidly set up and design your own website, preferable to paying someone else large sums of money to do this for you. Once up and running, it is possible to use software to engineer it appearing in searches.

6. Appropriability

Appropriability refers to the framework of legal and economic conditions that affect your ability to carry out business. This is dependent on two factors: protectability and freedom to operate. Protectability is the degree to which you can prevent competitors copying and exploiting your ideas. This protects your revenues and market share. Freedom to operate is the degree to which you can carry out your idea without copying or infringing the rights of other inventors or businesses, ideally without giving too much away.

Intellectual property (IP) results from the expression of an idea. It may be a brand, an invention, a design or a song and can be bought or sold. Patents (Patents Act 1977) protect the features and processes that make things work and allow inventors to profit from their inventions. Patents can last up to 20 years but are subject to annual review and fee. Patents are territorial. This means that if granted in the UK, it will only apply to the UK.

Copyright is an automatic right that protects written and recorded material, by writing the © symbol with your name and date. It prevents your work being copied or reproduced and can last for life plus 70 years. As the owner of the copyright, you have the right to license, sell or transfer the copyright to someone else.

Trademarks are symbols, like logos and brand names that distinguish different goods in the market place. Branding is discussed more in Chapter 7 on marketing. The rights to trademarks last forever, although they are reviewed every 10 years. No one else can use your trademark without your permission. Of note, registering a company name at Companies House does not automatically mean that the name will be accepted as a trademark.

7. Entrepreneurial team

This is one of the most critical factors for success in setting up your own business. In the experience of the authors, and the case study in Box 13.1, combining the efforts of complimentary skills in a partnership not only makes you more likely to be successful but also provides support and hopefully fun along the way. At a later stage, hiring employees requires yet more bureaucracy but allows you to delegate and focus on developing the strategic vision for the business that is crucial for longevity. Chapter 7 discusses teamwork in more detail.

SOCIAL ENTERPRISES

> Social enterprise is the great institutional innovation of our times.
>
> *David Cameron (2007)*

> Social enterprise offers radical new ways of operating for public benefit. By combining a strong public service ethos with business acumen, we can open up the possibility of entrepreneurial organisations – highly responsive to customers and with the freedom of the private sector – but which are driven by a commitment to public benefit rather than purely maximizing profits for shareholders.
>
> *Tony Blair (2002)*

The final section of this chapter focuses on a relatively new but fast growing business approach, called social enterprise. The Department for Trade and Industry describes a social enterprise as 'A business with primarily social objectives whose surpluses are principally reinvested for that purpose in the business or the community, rather than being driven by the need to maximise profit for shareholders and owners'.

However, many have broader definitions for social enterprises:

> Any innovative action that individuals, organisations, or networks conduct to enhance or reconfigure existing institutional arrangements to address the inadequate provision, or unequal distribution, of social and environmental goods.

It is clear though that three core elements define a social enterprise. First, that they are structured as effective businesses; thus there is a real requirement to make a profit, unlike a charity. Next, they need to be innovative; either they are addressing an old problem in a new way or because they are creating a new service or product. An example of the former is Jamie Oliver's restaurant enterprise Fifteen. While restaurants themselves are not new, what was new was that those serving and cooking the food were learning a skill that they might otherwise never have had an opportunity to do. A further example of the latter might be Grameen Bank and microfinance. The final core facet is that they need to clearly make a difference to society.

Perhaps the reason for the lack of complete agreement on definition is the novelty of social enterprises. Social enterprises grew in the UK in the early 1990s. By 2001, the government had sufficiently realised the merit of social enterprises to modernise the third sector and make it a fit partner for social reform. An investment fund for startup social enterprises was set up with an initial injection of cash of around £100 million. The year 2001 also saw the DTI set up the social enterprise unit and in 2006 the Cabinet Office developed the Office of the Third Sector with its own minister.

The growth from humble beginning is astounding. The Annual Survey of Small Businesses from 2006–07 which is government sponsored, ascertained that there are an estimated 62000 social enterprises in the UK, contributing £24 billion GVA (Gross Value Added) to the UK economy. More recently, the State of Social Enterprise Survey found that social enterprises were twice as confident of future growth than equivalent small to medium for profits. This is not false optimism. More than half of social enterprises have increased their profit from the year before, compared to their equivalent sized for profits, where only a quarter have done so. Perhaps most excitingly of all the social enterprise movement seems to be reforming society in a way that it could not have dreamed of: double the number of these companies are female driven, compared to the equivalent for profits, and nearly four times as many women sit as board members on social enterprises than on FTSE 100 companies.

Interestingly, the social enterprise movement seems to have caught the public imagination. Not just because of the number of new such companies. Thirty-five per cent of all entrepreneurs who have started a company in the last three months in the UK are taking part in a social enterprise. Furthermore 45% of people who set up social enterprises did so primarily to 'put something back into the community'. The trend that has led to the rise of social enterprise is distilled in the definition of a 'gift economy', or Generation G:

> Generation G captures the growing importance of 'generosity' as a leading societal and business mindset. As consumers are disgusted with greed and its dire consequences for the economy . . . the need for more generosity beautifully coincides with the ongoing (and pre-recession) emergence of an online-fuelled culture of individuals who share, give, engage, create and collaborate in large numbers.
>
> (Trendwatching, 2009)

Perhaps more importantly, the public wants to work for a social enterprise more than government, a business or indeed a charity. The overwhelming majority of people want social enterprises to run their public services. This is a remarkable achievement in less than 20 years, with important implication for healthcare provision and an achievement that the UK has spearheaded.

Social enterprises sit along a spectrum, shown in Figure 13.2. At one extreme is the for-profit company – often legally set up as a limited company. Moving towards the social benefit side is the for-profit company with a strong corporate social responsibility (CSR) arm. Whilst many argue whether CSR really exists or whether it is simply disguised marketing, there is a still a net direct benefit to society from this approach, albeit where CSR works best directed along the lines of the company strategy. An example might be a technology firm funding education and training in engineering.

The next step is the public–private partnership. Here, organisations maintain their classic form but actively choose to work together to the benefit of both sides. An example of such a partnership might be drug companies working with governments in the developing world. Social enterprises sit squarely in the middle. The benefit of straddling this spectrum is essentially a best of both worlds approach. Social enterprises have the good will of a not for profit or charity, but the business-like approach of a for profit. They have the access to capital of a for profit but the heart of a not for profit. Bridging this divide is not only a perfect place to enhance society but is also theoretically a place where innovation can occur.

Next are the cooperatives and mutual societies, e.g. the old style building societies. The next step would be a true not for profit, i.e. company limited by guarantee. Their rules of association ensure that there are no shareholders. In the event of dissolution, monies are given to pre-destined charitable efforts.

Next are charities, overseen by the Charities Commission in the UK. Finally, purely voluntary organisations. Whilst this spectrum might simplify and explain, the reality is murkier: many charities increasingly have profit making arms that give their surpluses to the charity. Equally, some social enterprises pay dividends to shareholders. As a result of this murkiness, there is considerable effort at present going into developing regulation or kite marking to clarify who is or is not a social enterprise.

Perhaps this murkiness is in part the problem of defining social good. This is perhaps the most challenging aspect of the social enterprise. The challenge comes because if the third facet is to be in keeping with the first then the social good needs to be able to be proven in a clear business manner. To a certain extent, the reporting routes are defined by the governance structure – but this sets the minimum standard. Thus there are currently a number of options being used. First, simply using the usual accounts or reports filed at Companies House or with the Charity Commission to show that money has not been incorrectly appropriated. Second, using Social Return on Investment (SROI). In essence, this approach seeks to put a financial value on the social benefit occurring and combines this with the profit made to give a bottom

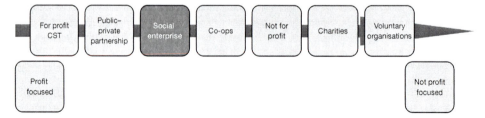

FIGURE 13.2 Social enterprises based on work of Alex Nicholls, Saïd Business School

line benefit in monetary terms. By converting good to money it allows comparison across social enterprises and indeed to other for profits.

The third option is for those social enterprises choosing to be incorporated as Community Interest Companies (CIC). This route was set up in 2004 under legislation and is a clear signal to the outside world of the approach of the company (it does not prohibit equity or capital raising but clear limits are put in place). Under this approach, a Community Interest Report (CIC34) has to be filed alongside the usual Companies House reports. This document details those aspects of the company that might require additional focus, e.g. how much directors have been paid, and therefore is overseen by a special regulator within Companies House. Another option is enhanced social audit. Here, the social actions at the heart of a company's structure are explored in a qualitative fashion. Nicholls has coined the term 'blended value accounting' to describe the spectrum of reporting of social and financial gain that has been described here.

The social enterprise model lends itself well to healthcare. In fact, the majority of social enterprise according to the DTIs 2005 survey is in health and social care (33%). One of the best-known UK health social enterprises is Turning Point, which has been providing specialist care for over 40 years. Turning Point specialises in services for substance misuse, mental health issues and learning disability. All of its profits are reinvested back into improving and providing services for people that need them most – in mental health, learning disability, substances misuse and for employment.

Turning Point neatly summaries a rationale for why the social enterprise movement has caught on and the role it can play in social reform. By existing as a social enterprise and clearly defining itself as a business with a desire to do good, but governed by strict financial and social regulations, yet free to seek capital to grow, Turning Point is able to signal that it is serious, efficient and reliable. The government has responded to this and to the public desire for social enterprises to run services. The introduction of World Class Commissioning (DH, 2007) has facilitated the growth of Turning Point, as Primary Care Trust (PCT). Commissioners have been able to choose preferred providers.

SUMMARY

Entrepreneurs will always identify opportunities in the environment around them. Looking ahead, it seems likely that competition will play an increasing role in the UK healthcare system. This provides an opportunity for clinicians to step up and lead top-quality services for patients, as doctorpreneurs.

In addition to covering the new world of social enterprise, this chapter provides practical advice about entrepreneurship and innovation. At present, there is limited encouragement and opportunity to nurture or value doctorpreneurial talent within the NHS. Being entrepreneurial requires being creative and bold enough to step outside of the mainstream.

Doing an MBA can provide the structure and confidence to support individuals who are drawn to do just this. Setting up your own business is not easy but the rewards are all yours, for the creating and the taking!

FURTHER READING

Branson R (2009). *Business Stripped Bare: adventures of a global entrepreneur*. London: Virgin Books.

Christensen CM, Grossman JH, Hwang J (2009). *The Innovator's Prescription: a disruptive solution for health care*. New York: McGraw-Hill Professional.

Community Interest Companies. www.cicregulator.gov.uk/

The Companies House. www.companieshouse.gov.uk/

Crisp N (2010). *Turning the World Upside Down: the search for global health in the 21st century*. London: The Royal Society of Medicine Press.

Enterprise UK. *Britain's got ambition: Virgin Media and Enterprise UK team up to unlock the UK's entrepreneurial spirit*. Available at: www.enterpriseuk.org/news/2010/03/12/britains_got_ambition_virgin_media_and_enterprise_uk_team_up_to_unlock_the_uks_entrepreneurial_spirit (accessed 20 June 2010).

HM Revenue and Customs. www.hmrc.gov.uk/index.htm

Moore G (1998). *Crossing the Chasm: marketing and selling technology products to mainstream customers*. Oxford: Capstone.

New Economics Foundation (2008). *Measuring Value: a guide to social return on investment*. 2nd ed. London: New Economics Foundation. Available at: www.proveandimprove.org/new/tools/sroi.php (accessed 20 June 2010).

Nicholls A, editor (2006). *Social Entrepreneurship: new models of sustainable social change*. Oxford: Oxford University Press.

Nicholls A (2009). 'We do good things, don't we? Blended value accounting in social entrepreneurship. *Accounting, Organizations and Society*; **34**: 755–69.

The Social Enterprise Coalition. www.socialenterprise.org.uk/

The Social Enterprise Coalition. *The State of Social Enterprises 2009*. Available at: www.socialenterprise.org.uk/data/files/stateofsocialenterprise2009.pdf (accessed 20 June 2010).

The SROI Network. www.sroi-uk.org/

CHAPTER 14

Strategy: plotting a path in healthcare

What do you want to achieve or avoid? The answers to this question
are objectives. How will you go about achieving your desired results?
The answer to this you can call strategy.

William E Rothschild

INTRODUCTION

Strategy is a word du jour. It is banded around and used to explain a variety of concepts, yet rarely is time taken to identify what it is and why it matters, particularly
for healthcare. This chapter lays out some of the ideas that make up strategy and
considers how this applies to the NHS. Through shedding light on these elements,
it is hoped that intrigue will be piqued and clinicians will become more engaged in
the strategic development of elements of healthcare.

To enable an abstract construct to be more readily understandable, concepts that
surround strategy will be examined at the hospital level. At present, many hospitals
are facing merger or closure or at least removal of some services. This chapter provides a framework for considering how to think about these issues. But strategy has
an effect at many more levels. Government health strategy has a profound effect on
frontline staff, as does wider public policy.

WHAT IS STRATEGY?

Strategy is 'a plan of action designed to achieve a particular goal' (Wikipedia). In the
corporate world, this translates into corporate strategy. This dictates which industry
a business should be in and how the business should be organised to compete well
within the chosen industry.

Much of business thinking around strategy looks at the former. The guru of strategy, Michael Porter of Harvard Business School, is renowned for his work in this area.
His five (or more recently six) forces for examining whether and how to enter a market have reached mythical status. In healthcare, examining which industry or market
to be in is slightly less relevant. Or at least it was less relevant. However, the recent
introduction of market mechanisms into the English healthcare economy, Chapter 8,
has made the market attractive to new entrants. Thus, organisations like Care UK or
Circle, would have had to use these or similar techniques to identify if entering the

healthcare market was rational and profitable. Equally, within the market of health-care they would have needed to examine where their niche might lie.

Consider a hypothetical company, Cure. A doctor, an ex-management consultant and the former head of strategy for a multi-national retail business, founded Cure. They are pondering whether to tender for contracts in the NHS. They decide to use Porter's five original forces to examine if, in the broadest possible terms, healthcare is worth dabbling into further, or if they should stick with their current business operations, which might be for example, veterinary medicine. The five forces are rivalry, entry threat, buyer power, supplier power, and substitutability. For Cure, the entry threat may be low if the government is trying to encourage new providers of care; as it is a new market there is limited rivalry and indeed the only substitute is the NHS. The issue for Cure is that there is limited supplier power; the buyer, i.e. the government, calls the shots. Thus Cure is able to think about progressing to a more detailed analysis of the market and the exact segment they might wish to inhabit, for example, running an acute hospital.

Business strategy is not divorced from corporate strategy, as it is essential to understand the market to compete well. However, business strategy focuses more on how the company or organisation can adapt and position themselves to max-imise their share of the market. These words may not seem relevant to healthcare in England. Yet virtually every region is currently seeing hospitals merge or face the threat of loss of services. In part, this is driven by evidence-based medicine. For exam-ple, evidence that regional trauma centres produce better outcomes, in part driven by safety demands linked to working hours, makes split sites unsustainable. Thus hospitals negotiating this choppy water do indeed need to understand their market and where their particular niche may lie, or alternatively accept that the good of those they serve is best enacted through merger or closure of services.

This highlights a core issue with strategy: that of who the strategy is designed for. In the business world it is clear that the strategy is designed to maximise shareholder value. In the public sector it is more complex. However, ultimately in a system funded by the public it must be the public value that is sought. Whilst organisations may choose to act in their best interest this needs to align with the public best interest. At times, this situation may only be clarified by external review. Complications may arise because of the conflict as to whether the local patients' opinion matters more than that of the general public, i.e. if local residents want the hospital or service to remain open, but value for money arguments dictate that closure makes more sense, what – and who – should win out?

If we return to St Anywhere Hospital, this stands in a region where it is clear from multiple reviews that there are too many district general hospitals (DGHs) in the vicinity. The question arises as to which should downgrade and become a local hospi-tal and which should upgrade into the expanding local acute hospital. This decision is made beyond the remit of the hospital. However, the hospital can position itself, by understanding the local market forces, to be in the best place for it and those it serves. Thus, the hospital may be able to demonstrate that it has strong market pene-tration, or that it has created an integrated health economy by tendering and winning provision of primary care services. (However, there are risks to moving beyond the core line of business. Much of the strategy literature around whether diversification is a good or bad idea is divided. The answer seems to be that it depends on multiple factors including the industry, the company and the timing, amongst other factors.) These initiatives might give the hospital the strategic influence to turn a decision.

This example also identifies that strategy is the blueprint. Much of the success of a strategy revolves around tactics and the action used to achieve a specific objective. As well as St Anywhere defining and enacting a broad strategy, it might also work to achieve its goal of becoming the local acute hospital (believing that this best serves the public) through tactical means. For example, if the hospital departments have an international or national reputation and this is clearly articulated, this might be a protective mechanism. Similarly, if the hospital is in a marginal seat and politicians can be convinced that the survival of the hospital is the desire of the local public, this too might influence advocacy for the hospital and perhaps also the outcome.

At the end of the day, strategy is just a document: what makes a strategy live and breathe is how this is expressed and what difference this makes. Convention does this through the values, mission, vision statement and set of objectives (some underline these with core values). The values are the heuristic patterns that the organisation wishes to engender. The vision outlines where the organisation aspires to be and what they want to be known for. The mission statement clarifies what needs to be done to achieve this. The objectives need to be measurable targets against which success can be judged. All too often there is blurring of these headings and poorly framed commitments. The best place to start when formulating a strategy is with the values of the organisation. From this flows the mission, hence the vision and then ultimately the mechanism to achieve this.

Trawling through companies outside of healthcare, memorable examples of visions include:

➤ Disney: 'We create happiness by providing the finest in entertainment for people of all ages, everywhere'.

➤ Apple: 'To produce high-quality, low cost, easy to use products that incorporate high technology for the individual. We are proving that high technology does not have to be intimidating for noncomputer experts'.

➤ Google: 'To make the world's information universally accessible and useful'.

➤ CIA: 'We will provide knowledge and take action to ensure the national security of the United States and the preservation for American life and ideals'.

In the hospital setting in the UK, an example of such a vision might be that of University College London Hospital (UCLH). 'UCLH is committed to delivering top quality patient care, excellent education and world class research'.

This vision is then expressed as 10 strategic goals:

1 Deliver excellent clinical outcomes
2 Improve patient safety
3 Deliver high quality patient experience
4 Deliver waiting time targets
5 Achieve sustainable financial health
6 Develop and enable staff
7 Progress strategic developments

8   Work with partners to improve patient pathways
9   Develop world class Research and Development and excellent education
10 Develop Governance and Risk Management Strategy.

UCLH VISION, AND GOALS

Each goal has sub-goals, each of which is specific, time-constrained and highly measureable. UCLH has adopted one style of strategy. Sharp, a healthcare provider in San Diego, California, presents another. Their mission statement is shown in Box 14.1 below:

BOX 14.1 Sharp

Mission statement

It is our mission to improve the health of those we serve with a commitment to excellence in all that we do. Our goal is to offer quality care and programs that set community standards, exceed patients' expectations and are provided in a caring, convenient, cost-effective and accessible manner.

Vision and Values

Sharp HealthCare's vision is to be the best health system in the universe. Sharp will attain this position by transforming the healthcare experience through a culture of caring, quality, service, innovation and excellence. Sharp will be recognized by employees, physicians, patients, volunteers and the community as the best place to work, the best place to practice medicine and the best place to receive care. Sharp is known as an excellent community citizen embodying an organisation of people working together to do the right thing every day to improve the health and well being of those we serve.

Sharp's core values are integrity, caring, innovation and excellence.

This serves to introduce a further point about strategies and their communication. Sharp, recent winners of the prestigious Presidential Award, the Baldrige Award for Quality, chose specifically to create a stretch goal: 'Sharp HealthCare's vision is to be the best health system in the universe'. Sharp set themselves a challenging target! Not content with being the best in the USA, they are competing with alien life forms no less. But the underlying statement in these bold words is clear. Sharp are not afraid of challenge. They desire to be up there with the best and are willing to set out their goals visibly in the public domain. This is as inspiring as it must be challenging.

Both strategies are dynamic rather than static. They show an understanding of the need to adapt to changing external environments.

Organisations use different methods to develop strategies. One way is to use scenarios for the future and to develop independent strategies to meet each of these futures. In healthcare, scenario planning and establishing the different options is often highly complex. For St Anywhere it might be that one scenario is for a review by the SHA and a decision to downgrade to a local hospital. The second option might be to become the local acute hospital and the third might be a merger with the adjacent DGH. Each scenario requires unique features, e.g. for the second option there might need to be additional capital expenditure on angioplasty suites. Some companies choose to create a strategy that will allow them to jump between these scenarios, i.e. a very flexible approach. However, the problem with this is that the strategy is less honed to individual outcomes. Where there are clues as to which scenario is more likely, it may be advantageous to focus on that scenario, whilst acknowledging and having a guide for dealing with the others, should they occur.

Ultimately what each of these strategies is doing is playing to the organisation's strength: for Google it is information accessibility; for Disney it is making people happy; for St Anywhere it might be that they provide a range of high quality services close to home. These are the organisation's competitive (or in the public sector – comparative) advantages. There are many ways to identify this. One is to look at the organisation's resources and capabilities and use this to identify the core competencies, using a SWOT analysis. Another is to look outside and ask users what they value most about a company. For the Ritz Carlton, this might be high quality individualised care, for Apple it might be innovative easy-to-use products that are highly reliable and look sleek. Porter identifies that companies can differentiate themselves in two underlying ways: on cost leadership or differentiation (i.e. either do it cheaper or better). For healthcare organisations where price competitions are difficult mainly due to the tariff, the key is therefore to do it better.

Perhaps though the fundamental element of strategy is alignment. Whilst it is of course important for organisations to express their strategy, if the strategy of an organisation is divorced from the actions of those who work for the organisation, then the strategy is unlikely to be successful.

An organisation that fully embodies how success can be generated by ensuring that those working in an organisation live and breathe the strategy is the previously discussed Mayo Clinic in the US. The Mayo's mission is clear: 'Mayo Clinic will provide the best care to every patient every day through integrated clinical practice, education and research'. What speaks loudest and what every employee from the janitor to the CEO will tell you is how this is to be achieved, through the guiding principle of the Mayo Clinic for over 100 years: 'The needs of the patient come first'.

This is inculcated into every part of the Mayo from day one of induction where new employees role play scenarios from the past history of the Mayo, to the boardroom where tactical decisions are often considered by asking what serves the patient best. It is this unending pursuit that makes the organisation great. Everything from physician pay through to governance arrangements are aligned with the strategic belief that the Mayo can move forward, be it opening new clinics or expanding into community care, and can do so successfully without compromising revenue or quality of care to always put the needs of the patient first.

SUMMARY

This chapter has stressed the importance of strategy. It is worth ending by remembering the story of Honda's market entry into the US motorbike industry. When Honda tried to break into the US market, its sale force attempted in vain to sell large bikes.

To enable them to so do they travelled around the country on small bikes. They failed to sell their original product but the small bikes became a sensation. This story leads to perhaps two questions: first, is strategy real or is it a posthoc rationalisation? And second, is strategy the be all and end all? Perhaps the answer to the first lies in the words of a renowned Oxbridge College President: 'when I stopped doing things for my CV I moved onto doing things for my Obituary'. To the outsider, obituaries are linear stories of a life, where it may seem that a strategy or direction can be elucidated. In reality, for most, life is much more about a series of sliding doors moments. The answer to the second is perhaps that a strategy allows you to be able to see the opportunities because it enables the organisation to run smoothly in the main.

FURTHER READING

Baldrige National Quality Program. www.baldrige.nist.gov/Contacts_Profiles.htm

Berry LL, Seltman KD (2008). *Management Lessons from Mayo Clinic.* New York: McGraw Hill.

Besanko D, Dranove D, Shanley M, *et al.* (2007). *Economics of Strategy.* 4th ed. Hoboken, NJ: John Wiley & Sons, Inc.

Business Resource Software. Mission statement. www.businessplans.org/mission.html

Grant RM (2008). *Contemporary Strategy Analysis.* 6th ed. Oxford: Blackwell Publishing.

The Mayo Clinic. Mayo's mission. www.mayoclinic.org/about/missionvalues.html

McCay L, Jonas S (2009). *A Junior Doctor's Guide to the NHS.* London: Medical Directorate of the Department of Health. Available at: http://group.bmj.com/group/affinity-and-society-publishing/NHS%20Guide.pdf (accessed 22 April 2010)

Pettigrew A, Ferlie E, McKee L (1992). *Shaping Strategic Change.* London: Sage Publications Ltd.

Porter M (January 2008). The five competitive forces that shape strategy. *Harvard Business Review*; 79: 79–93.

Porter ME, Olmsted Teisberg E (2006). *Redefining Health Care.* Boston, MA: Harvard Business School Press.

SHARP: San Diego's Health Care Leader. Mission, vision and values. www.sharp.com/choose-sharp/mission-vision-values.cfm

University College London Hospitals (UCLH). About UCLH. www.uclh.nhs.uk/About+UCLH/Mission+and+objectives/

SECTION 4

Flying with an MBA

Most gulls don't bother to learn more than the simplest facts of flight; how to get from shore to food and back again. For most gulls it is not flying that matters, but eating. For this gull, though, it was not eating that mattered, but flight.

Richard Bach, Jonathan Livingston Seagull

Doing an MBA and having ambition beyond your clinical training will, at times, seem threatening to your medical colleagues and peers. Jonathan Livingston Seagull is an inspiring story about seeking a higher vision and soaring to reach it. An MBA broadens horizons and abilities, leading to opportunities for individuals to fly.

The final two chapters of this book consider career opportunities open to clinicians with MBAs to soar in the NHS and beyond.

FURTHER READING

Bach R (1970). *Jonathan Livingston Seagull: a story*. London: Element Books.

Lee F (2004). *If Disney Ran Your Hospital: 9½ things you would do differently*. Bozeman, MT: Second River Healthcare Press.

CHAPTER 15

To MBA or not to MBA: how is it likely to affect a career in the NHS?

> The leadership instinct you are born with is the backbone. You develop the funny bone and the wishbone that go with it.
>
> *Elaine Agather*

In Chapter 2 the argument is made that qualifications in management, and amongst them MBAs, are ever more seen as important badges, in an increasingly competitive world. This chapter looks at how MBAs may benefit the NHS. First, there is an examination of some of the leadership roles that doctors play. This is then followed by an examination of the role of the MBA in leadership and management.

LEADERSHIP OPPORTUNITIES

Whilst in many industries leadership is pretty much focused on running an organisation, e.g. a company or conglomerate, healthcare offers much greater breadth of such roles. Although many clinicians have little contact with their executive teams, most are aware if by name only of their CEO, and maybe even Chair; they are eminently more likely to recognise their Medical Director. Clinicians are also aware albeit maybe vaguely of the college presidents, although the increasing number of colleges may mean that knowledge is confined to their specialty. Similarly, clinicians may well have a vague inkling of the head of the BMA and maybe even sub-sections such as the head of the GP committee. Perhaps less well known are other leadership roles: roles within Arms Length Bodies, the Department of Health (DH) and other governmental departments.

This section examines briefly a few such roles. The implication should not be taken that these roles require degrees in management. Rather that these are leadership roles that those who are interested in such areas might aspire to. Furthermore there are many roles within the healthcare sphere that are not currently occupied by those with a medical background, but this does not mean that in the future this need continue to be the case.

For an increasing number of doctors, management is a powerful route to redefining the healthcare system that they belong to. In the past, changing healthcare through policy has been the domain of public health physicians. Public health physicians act locally and nationally to help define laws, regulations and policies that determine how healthcare is delivered. Public health doctors can be found in a diverse variety of settings, including Primary Care Trusts (PCTs), Strategic Health Authorities (SHAs), Arms Length Bodies such as the Health Protection Agency (HPA), charities, and local and national government.

Overseeing and supporting public health physicians involved in regional work is one of the many roles of the Chief Medical Officer for England (CMO). The position of the CMO was created in 1855, to help deal with the cholera epidemics sweeping the country. The first CMO was Sir John Simon, and the current is Dame Sally Davies, following the retirement of Sir Liam Donaldson in May 2010.

Over time the role has evolved, such that there are now four regional CMOs – one for each devolved region. In addition, the CMO for England serves as the Chief Medical Advisor to the UK Government. In this capacity the CMO is called upon to produce diverse policy documents, some of which lead directly to adoption by government; others serve to chart potential future directions for policy, and stimulate essential public debate. Debate that is clearly perceived by the public and professionals to be independent and evidence-based. An example of policy that led to legislation is *Good Doctor, Safer Patients*, written in the light of the public medical scandals and in an attempt to restore public confidence in the medical profession. It set out clear expectations for doctors. This led to the introduction of both secondary and primary legislation (*Trust, assurance and safety: the regulation of the medical profession*). *Stem cell research: medical progress with responsibility*, framed the debate around stem cells, and permitted the UK to be in the vanguard for ethical clarity with respect to this new field of science. Perhaps though, the recently retired occupant of this role is best known for his championing of the nascent field of patient safety, through a series of reports and regular coverage in his influential annual reports.

The CMO also serves as a permanent secretary to the Department of Health. In this role she manages three departments within the department: Research and Development, Health Improvement and Protection and Regional Public Health Groups. She works closely with co-permanent secretaries, currently Hugh Taylor and the NHS Chief Executive, Sir David Nicholson, to ensure the smooth running and strategy of the Department of Health. On a day-to-day basis this means sitting on both the NHS Management Board and the Departmental Board.

The CMO also acts as a unique interface between government and the public. Sir Liam was widely recognised as independent and authoritative, as seen by the extent of his media involvement in public health issues such as pandemic flu. He provided clear, accurate, non-sensational information both directly to the public through media interviews and for the media through briefings. His outward-facing role also extended to professionals. Whilst there are many medical leaders, few have the access to the internal mechanisms of government that the role of CMO does.

The exact domains of the CMO within the Department of Health have waxed and waned over many years. With the recent theme of increasing independence for the NHS, the role of Medical Director for the NHS was re-created. The current occupant of this role is Professor Sir Bruce Keogh. This is both an operational and strategic role, with dual reporting lines to the CMO, and the NHS CEO, since the post holder is also a deputy CMO. The role provides an oversight to internal departments such as those managing clinical quality and safety as well as external bodies such as the

National Institute for Health and Clinical Excellence (NICE) and the National Patient Safety Agency (NPSA). The NHS Medical Director is also a powerful point of contact for fellow local NHS medical directors, thereby helping to connect the department to the frontline of care.

Within the Department of Health, doctors hold a number of other key positions. First, the Director of Research and Development, currently Dame Sally Davies. This director is responsible both for defining the research agenda through the newly established National Institute for Health Research and the Policy Research Programme. This department also oversees academic medical training programmes such as the Academic Clinical Fellowships.

The newly created post of Director of Medical Education is presently occupied by Patricia Hamilton. This role was developed to oversee Modernising Medical Careers implementation and strengthened in the light of the Tooke Report. Dr Hamilton reports to the NHS Medical Director as do a number of other senior medics within the department. This group of doctors, commonly known as the 'Tsars', are the National Clinical Directors, the first of whom stepped into post 10 years ago. Today there are more than 10 such directors covering emergency preparedness, pandemic flu, cancer, heart disease, diabetes, renal disease, trauma, transplantation, mental health, primary care, health and work, and maternal and child health. Their role originally developed to permit clinical oversight of the development of the National Service Frameworks – strategies for improvement for areas such as cancer and cardiac care. Today their role is varied, maintaining policy input and spearheading change, as well as acting as key coordinators for their disciplines across government. As an example, Sheila Shribman, the National Clinical Director for Children, Young People and Maternity Services, coordinates approaches to improving children's medical care across departments, including the Department for Children, Schools and Families (DCSF), Cabinet Office and Department of Health.

Whilst these doctors serve as leaders both within the Department of Health, and to the wider profession and public, there are also a number of doctors who work at the heart of policy development and implementation. As an example, Professor David Salisbury leads the Immunisation Team. A paediatrician by background, Professor Salisbury has contributed enormously to the creation of our current vaccination programmes and to the emergency response to new threats such as pandemic flu.

Similarly there are a large number of doctors who spend time either seconded to the department or working for the department, for example, chairing working groups. One of the most high profile recent examples of this is Lord Ara Darzi of Denham, who spent two years as Parliamentary Under-Secretary of State (Lords). A practising surgeon, he devoted his time in the Department of Health to both day-to-day ministerial work and spearheading a review of the NHS. His recommendation delivered as *High Quality Care for all: the next stage review final report* has been a powerful blueprint for a new phase of NHS development, with a focus on the quality of care (Chapter 3). This report created a new chapter in clinician involvement in policy making, as thousands of clinicians willingly gave up their time to participate in the development of both local and national strategies for clinical pathways.

To many clinicians, the Department of Health feels like a black box that is unknown and slightly intimidating. The valiant work of clinicians who step from the world of active clinical practice into this 'other world' is helping to create policies more in tune with real need, and are practical, actionable and more accepted by clinicians and patients. Clinician involvement in the policy process is very much defined by individual enthusiasm, professional acceptance and governmental attitude. At present, all three are aligned such that there are real opportunities to play a role in this process, whether through local Strategic Health Authorities, or centrally. Opportunities exist at present to act as a powerful voice for health beyond even the Department of Health with the recent appointment of a CMO at the Department of Transport.

Similarly, most Arms Length Bodies have a core team of medics, for example: Health Protection Agency (HPA), NICE, and the NPSA. While many of these clinicians work part-time for these bodies and maintain clinical practice alongside this work, some move over entirely.

For some, this has been a progression from leadership roles within trusts, for others their careers have been developed within these bodies, learning the specific skills that the institutions demand. These career paths may not suit all, but it is important to be aware that the opportunities exist and to encourage younger clinicians to consider whether these roles appeal for them.

DO YOU NEED AN MBA (OR EQUIVALENT) TO DO THESE ROLES?

Today, doctors with MBAs in the NHS are a tiny minority; even those who are currently in leadership roles rarely have such a degree. Those who do have made conscious individual choices to subject themselves to at least a year of gruelling and exhilarating training. Moreover, save for a few isolated schemes and the occasional institution willing to co-fund, most of those with MBAs have incurred a financial penalty to undertake this degree. Thus those who have done so have clearly seen merit in advance, and in the main, upon completion (if MBA feedback and rankings are to be believed).

With such scarce evidence, due to the paucity of individuals with MBAs, especially in senior positions, it is hard to identify how an MBA actively alters career paths. As with many training experiences it is also tricky to untangle the cause and effect: would those who choose MBAs have achieved anyway, or is it the MBA that led to the success?

One way to start to examine the benefit of MBAs is perhaps to look to other healthcare systems where clinicians play a very active role in leadership and management. The Mayo Clinic in the US is world renowned for many reasons, not least for having a physician as CEO and President since it began. The clinical leadership at the Mayo has much to teach but intriguingly it has never, to date, had a CEO with a formal management degree, including an MBA. Instead, those who have led the Mayo have learnt their skills and knowledge from experience and not just their own experience. Rather from their first tentative steps into the world of management they are paired, with an administrator. The administrator's role is to facilitate the leadership and management decisions of the clinicians. Thus the clinician can focus on idea development and human relationships whilst the administrator converts the ideas into businesses cases and strategic plans, training the doctor as they go.

It is clear that there is strength in this model, with each profession playing to their spheres of knowledge and harnessing the combination for synergistic effect. But this comes at a price for the administrator – a price they are willing to pay that they will not be the forward-facing leader, rather more the backroom facilitator. In this model, formal qualifications are less relevant. Furthermore, those clinicians chosen to grow through the ranks of leadership positions do so because of the strength of their clinical, research and teaching prowess rather than their management acumen. This helps maintain the respect of their colleagues when they do develop into these leadership roles. Most importantly, these roles are not dead ends. Most senior leadership roles at the Mayo are time limited and many clinicians go back after even the most senior posts to clinical duties that are equivalent to being a normal consultant, not even a divisional lead. Accompanying this logic is that the pay benefit of such a role is a modest 5–10%. This is sustained even when returning to practice. Thus leadership does not end the involvement in medicine nor constitute a divorce from it; rather it is simply one phase of a career, where those who have shown signs of aptitude contribute to the organisation in a way that others may not be able to or wish to.

For many, the practice at the Mayo is a nirvana – where clinical leadership and medical management should aim to be. Few organisations in the UK could point to a similar set up. Even where medics lead they do so by stepping outside of the normal medical career path and do so in a way that is almost inevitably unidirectional. Professor Chris Ham and colleagues, in a recent report, highlight these concerns (2010). One suggested route to minimising this might be to adopt the Danish system, where for every year out of clinical practice, a month of re-training is offered should the clinician want to return to the frontline CEO post. This has its attractions, particularly with changes to revalidation on the horizon. Of note, the US model does not include this. This is, in part, because the CEOs often remain able to do clinical work through their time as CEO. Ham *et al.* found that of the 22 UK medical CEOs interviewed, several were achieving this (some up to two days per week) but others felt time and responsibility did not and should not allow this.

Furthermore because of the very nature of unidirectionality, because it is a choice to seek this route rather than a bestowed honour, this step can often lead to a decrease rather than an increase in respect from colleagues. Ham *et al.* argues strongly that all too often stepping up is not valued by clinical colleagues. They also identify that for many who have chosen the medical CEO route it is because of a desire to help groups of patients, in addition to a slight sense of competition – if other non-medics can do it, why not them? This optimism however belies the fact that actually achieving such a role can be difficult, slightly less so if the clinician is appointed to the CEO role from within the organisation. Whilst it is important to note that the stories from Ham *et al.* show a clear sense of the roles being enjoyed, there is also a very potent sense of the burden and anxiety heightened by factors like the short tenure of CEOs as a group within the NHS. Equally, there are concerns about pay gaps between clinical colleagues and CEOs.

Perhaps it is because of these that, unlike the Mayo, medics in leadership roles have a history of either formal management qualifications like MBAs or indeed have stepped outside of healthcare – maybe into consulting, to gain the relevant experience, perhaps seeking confidence and recognition to allow movement into a future

NHS leadership position. Many believe that alongside the current active focus on training all in clinical leadership through their undergraduate and postgraduate training, funding should be available for interested parties to compete for full or part funding for managerial degrees – perhaps MBAs or healthcare management degrees (or even short courses in management).

There may indeed be a broader vision that needs to be aimed for in the UK, one which would help reassert a sense of professionalism and perhaps bridge the doctor–management divide. Surely the quest should be not for medics who are managers, but rather medics who are leaders with administrators by their side, walking step by step to help realise their vision – akin to the Mayo model. This desire for leading rather than managing is palpable through the words of current medical CEOs as transcribed and interpreted by Ham *et al.* This contentious viewpoint means a lot of changes. First, it means institutional nurturing of future leaders. Second, it means managers shifting their position to an administrative function, paired with clinicians. Third, it means changes to career structure such that leadership is not an end but simply a step along a career. Fourth, it means that those stepping up to these roles need to be people who excel at the core requirements for physicians – clinical work (including quality improvement), research and education. Finally it means altering remuneration packages, so that stepping into these roles does not dramatically increase salary, nor does stepping out decrease. Many of these ideas are mirrored by Ham *et al.* in their recommendations. This is not to say that clinicians who want to be actively involved in management cannot or are excluded from these roles, rather that these individuals are such that they might spend more of their careers in these leadership roles, for example as chairs of committees and/or divisional managers.

If such a vision is the end goal – where do MBAs fit in? The answer comes in part from a reality check. Achieving the vision above is not possible through national or even regional decrees. It will only occur within institutions – perhaps AHSC are the most likely environments to foster this innovation. It is unlikely to occur immediately, since nurturing those with potential, changing career routes, realigning managerial relations with clinicians, remuneration and professional respect is a slow and bureaucratically laboured process. There is anecdotal evidence that where steps are starting to occur in this direction the response has been impressive. One example of this is Service Line Management. In hospitals where this is actively functional, there has been pairing of clinicians with managers. These partnerships have helped to deliver autonomy, efficiency, productivity and perhaps most importantly have been morale boosting.

Achieving the whole package will only happen if individuals are committed to this as a route to more effective healthcare. It may be through doing degrees like MBAs that clinicians start to understand and look to other industries and other healthcare organisations, and start to see what works and what does not and start to share the vision outlined above, and most importantly have the skills to make it happen. MBAs may not be the solution to medical management or clinical leadership of the future in the NHS. However, they may be a supportive measure to getting the NHS to a vision such as that outlined earlier. They may be the confidence and skill boost that the pioneers require.

SUMMARY

This chapter has shared examples of roles within the NHS and the Department of Health for medics with MBAs, as well as learning from international best experience, models from the US and Denmark.

Medicine is perhaps the best example of how much can be learnt in classes and from books and yet how much more important understanding and wisdom comes from experience. Management study after management study shows that experience is superior training to course-based learning. Both are required but the art of medicine, as with the art of leadership or management, comes from role modelling, through overcoming frustrations and discovering pleasures that are experienced along the journey. An MBA may provide the catalyst but it is what individuals choose to do with them that will help to define the NHS of the future.

FURTHER READING

Berry LL, Seltman KD (2008). *Management Lessons from Mayo Clinic*. New York: McGraw Hill.

Department of Health (2000). *Stem Cell Research: medical progress with responsibility*. London: Department of Health. Available at: www.dh.gov.uk/en/Publicationsandstatistics/Publications/PublicationsPolicyAndGuidance/DH_4065084 (accessed 20 April 2010).

Department of Health (2006). *Good Doctors, Safer Patients: proposals to strengthen the system to assure and improve the performance of doctors and to protect the safety of patients*. London: Department of Health. Available at: www.dh.gov.uk/en/Publicationsandstatistics/Publications/PublicationsPolicyAndGuidance/DH_4137232 (accessed 20 April 2010).

Department of Health (2007). *Aspiring to Excellence Final Report of the Independent Inquiry into Modernising Medical Careers*. London: Department of Health. Available at: www.mmcinquiry.org.uk/draft.htm (accessed 20 April 2010).

Department of Health (2007). *Trust, Assurance and Safety: the regulation of health professionals*. London: Department of Health. Available at: www.dh.gov.uk/en/Publicationsandstatistics/Publications/PublicationsPolicyAndGuidance/DH_065946 (accessed 20 April 2010).

Department of Health (2008). *High Quality Care for all: the next stage review final report*. London: Department of Health. Available at: www.dh.gov.uk/en/Publicationsandstatistics/Publications/PublicationsPolicyAndGuidance/DH_085825 (accessed 20 April 2010).

Department of Health (2009). *150 years of the Annual Report of the Chief Medical Officer: on the state of public health 2008*. London: Department of Health. Available at: www.dh.gov.uk/en/Publicationsandstatistics/Publications/AnnualReports/DH_096206 (accessed 20 April 2010).

Ham C, Clark J, Spurgeon P, et al. (2010). *Medical Chief Executives in the NHS: facilitators and barriers to their career progression*. Warwick: NHS Institute for Improvement and Innovation.

McCay L, Jonas S (2009). *A Junior Doctor's Guide to the NHS*. London: Medical Directorate of the Department of Health. Available at: http://group.bmj.com/group/affinity-and-society-publishing/NHS%20Guide.pdf

Sheard S, Donaldson L (2005). *The Nation's Doctor*. Oxford: Radcliffe Publishing Ltd.

CHAPTER 16

Boundroids

> If you can imagine it, you can achieve it; if you can dream it, you can become it.
>
> *William Arthur Ward*

INTRODUCTION

Not all law students will become practising solicitors or barristers. Similarly for medicine, not all medical students will remain practising clinicians for the duration of their careers. Combining clinical experience with an MBA provides a strong platform to launch into a wide range of future career paths.

The preceding chapter considered potential career paths for doctors within the NHS and the Department of Health. This chapter considers career opportunities for medics with MBAs beyond the NHS. It is not an exhaustive list and the career categories discussed are not solely for those with MBAs. The aim of this chapter is to provide some initial ideas that may be of interest and warrant further exploration, either pre-, peri- or post-MBA.

As with all Masters Degrees, an MBA provides breadth of learning across all sectors of industry and society. It serves to broaden individual horizons and ambition. With an increasingly globalised market for talent, medics who do MBAs will not only be introduced to opportunities in sectors beyond healthcare but also to international opportunities. Recruiters frequent business schools to identify top talent, known as a 'milk round'. Doctors with MBAs will inevitably be among those that attract headhunters' attention.

Unlike medical school, much of the coursework for MBAs is carried out in allocated teams, working with individuals from a range of professional backgrounds and different countries. This develops bonds between individuals and provides a network of contacts for future collaboration. These relationships may also evolve in a Darwinian and innovative fashion into employment opportunities. The below areas of career opportunities are presented in alphabetical order. Where possible, case studies of medics with MBAs have been included, with permission.

ACADEMIC

Many medical specialties encourage high potential trainees to undertake MDs or PhDs alongside their clinical training. A higher research degree is particularly important for trainees who aspire to work in top teaching hospitals or have future academic career paths. Within management, the equivalent to a PhD is a DBA (Doctorate in Business Administration). An MBA acts as a gateway to this qualification. Doctors who do DBAs are rare but may aspire to an academic career, such as becoming a Chair in a Department of Healthcare Management, within a business school or university. Such positions could be combined with international advisory roles, for example at the Global Health Fund or the World Health Organization.

There are also academic roles for medics with commercial acumen to work alongside health economists in think tanks such as The King's Fund and the Nuffield Trust. Even if a full-time role in these organisations does not appeal, opportunities exist to become honorary fellows of academic institutions such as Judge Business School and Imperial College Business School. Maintaining an academic interest in healthcare management, in whatever future career path you choose, provides access to lectures and debates on key issues in healthcare policy as well as the opportunity to network, keep up to date with and – if desired – to publish academic articles with colleagues.

Academia relies on an ability to attract funding to survive. Therefore, an MBA is a desirable qualification for academics who aspire to lead departments, teams and co-ordinate research funding. There are also opportunities within medical education for medics with MBAs to be involved in publishing, running courses and conferences.

Box 16.1 illustrates the story of a medic with an MBA who has a leadership role at Cambridge Judge Business School.

BOX 16.1 The MBA changed my life

Jenny Dean, MB ChB MSc MBA
Executive Director, Centre for Health Leadership and Enterprise, Cambridge Judge Business School, 2010

The Cambridge MBA changed my life! It was quite an investment and not a little risk to take, but it was worth every penny; and I guess I made sure that I made the most of it to make it so. I wanted a well-balanced experience: some time out to consider career opportunities; build a diverse and high profile network; knowledge and skills to broaden my education; and a respected degree with a powerful brand – and those are exactly what I got.

The most powerful asset that I gained from my MBA, in addition to the strong brand, was the network that I started to build and invest in throughout my MBA and which continues to thrive and grow even more so today. This network has opened doors to me that I would otherwise not have been able to knock on. It led to my current role, returning to the same business school to establish the research Centre for Health Leadership & Enterprise; where it also enabled me to make significant progress almost immediately.

The knowledge and skills I developed during the MBA have also been instrumental in this role where I have used them to develop a strategy for the Centre, taking into account our best position in the market, understanding our 'customers' and how to engage our various

(continued)

---

stakeholders. Designing an effective business model for sustainability and undertaking the day-to-day accounts are also activities that, like the others, are relatively common sense, but have been made easier and more effective by learning useful frameworks and principles within which to undertake them. It's like learning how to take a patient history in a clear structured comprehensive format.

DOCTORPRENEUR

Mohammad Al-Ubaydli graduated as a doctor in 2000 and is currently doing a distance MBA at Robert Kennedy College, Switzerland. He describes a medical degree as 'a licence to do anything you want to in life'. Many clinicians fear the uncertainty of stepping away from the secure and predictable scaffolding of traditional medical hierarchy. However, for entrepreneurs – like Mohammad – stepping away from a traditional career path is a breeding ground for freedom and opportunity rather than fear.

In 2002, the NHS launched a national programme for IT (Information Technology) that excluded small innovative companies from securing contracts. Following this, Mohammad boldly decided to go to the US where he gained experience in publishing computer software, management consultancy and observed how Google and Microsoft were applying their technological prowess to projects in healthcare. Mohammad returned to the UK in 2008 when it became clear that the national programme for IT was in trouble. He then launched his company Patients Know Best, which provides secure personal health records, accessible by both patients and doctors. Mohammad believes that there is huge potential for medics with the ability to think laterally, combining technological, commercial and clinical know-how to disruptively innovate in healthcare. Mohammad has a pragmatic entrepreneurial approach to risk taking. His move to the US when the UK market was unreceptive for his ideas demonstrates resilience and opportunism, essential characteristics for success as a doctorpreneur.

HEALTH TECHNOLOGY

Why is it that most restaurants and cafes are able to take orders on handheld computers that communicate directly with the kitchen staff, yet clinicians in the NHS continue to keep patient histories, handwritten on paper medical notes and forms? To date, healthcare is patchy in its adoption of innovation and technology.

As set out at the beginning of this book, 17% of UK public spend is on healthcare (2009). Both the amount and proportion of spend on healthcare provision are set to rise. This means that all companies, including those in the technology field, are considering the relevance of their services to this growing market.

In large technology companies, such as Google and Cisco, there are specific healthcare departments. For others, specific healthcare departments and jobs may not yet exist. The best advice for medics with MBAs wanting to enter this sector is to find a company that you would like to work for, and send an email to set up a meeting. Waiting for your dream job to be advertised in the *BMJ* has a very low probability of occurrence. Instead, accept an entry-level job and demonstrate aptitude. Following a period of orientation and training, medics with MBAs are likely to rapidly fly into senior influential positions. But don't expect to enter at the senior level you aspire to. Initially like everyone else, you will need to demonstrate your value for money.

MANAGEMENT CONSULTANCY

> A management consultant is someone who will borrow your watch and use it to tell you the time.

While some may consider being a management consultant the last thing they would ever want to do, there is both benefit and opportunity in understanding how a management consultant operates. There is no better way to do this than to spend time being one. Both authors have learnt valuable lessons about pitching, client management, working under pressure and change management in healthcare through secondments working alongside management consultants. Although the demands of working as a management consultant can be ferocious, the rewards include corporate benefits packages (perks such as private gym membership, blackberries and company credit cards) added to notably higher salaries than those within the NHS. In addition to healthcare, management consultancy offers voyeuristic insights into the mechanics of a wide range of businesses.

The drawbacks of consultancy are that projects are often short-term. Ultimately, it is up to the client whether to follow the strategic advice you, as the management consultant, may be suggesting. Such compromises can be frustrating. However, consultancy work does provide a mechanism to experience working in many different areas of the healthcare economy at a strategic level. The network this generates is likely to lead to future career avenues. In addition, many former management consultants say that one of the most valuable assets they carry forward from being a management consultant is the alumni network.

In the UK, despite the recent recession, healthcare management consultancy is a healthily growing field. Entry to large management consultancies, such as BCG (Boston Consulting Group) and McKinsey & Company, is competitive. Thus, having an MBA will undoubtedly convey advantage and demonstrate ability at application and interview.

PHARMACEUTICAL INDUSTRY

There is ongoing controversy about the relationship between medics, evidence and the pharmaceutical industry. However, this industry provides a well-trodden career path for many medics who leave clinical practice. For these individuals, an MBA brings advantage to career progression and leadership roles, competing with non-medics for senior positions. For Dr Vinay Patroe, Director of Respiratory, UK Medical at GlaxoSmithKline, doing an MBA enabled him to understand the jargon associated with accounting and marketing. Through this, he was able to make sense of balance sheets and cash statements (*see* Chapter 9).

'An MBA is less about having the letters after your name. It is more about putting the learnings into action and showing an appreciation of what important business drivers are such that valuable activities are delivered excellently, one can be a great team member or leader and can also help others to perform and deliver to the best of their ability'.

Box 16.2 shares the experience of a pharmaceutical physician who completed an MBA at the University of Connecticut (2008) and describes the opportunities at entry level for medics into the pharmaceutical industry.

BOX 16.2 Overcoming the stigma of being
a physician in the pharma industry

Dr Ed Tucker, Vice President of Pharmacovigilance at Bayer Healthcare,
completed his MBA at the University of Connecticut (2008)

As a Physician, you have a clear and uniquely defining competency, which is greatly valued in many professional sectors. Therefore, a Masters in Business Administration (MBA) will rarely surpass the value of medical qualifications and will simply serve as an adjunct or an enhancement to your original talents. One exception is when a physician chooses to leave the medical sector and competes with scholars for occupations that require commercial or general business skills. Studying an MBA facilitates essential conversations with colleagues who are charged with responsibilities outside of the medical disciplines.

Physicians have potential careers in the Pharmaceutical industry through various means of entry and development, including medical support for clinical development (toxicology, pharmacology and late stage development); communication or medical affairs; regulatory; or patient safety and clinical risk management (Pharmacovigilance). Other opportunities exist in health outcomes research, commercial analytics, strategic business development, public communications and country/regional management. In addition, Physicians could consider entering the Financial Institutions as a Pharmaceutical Analyst (see below). The decision as to which discipline to choose relies on the baseline qualifications, competencies attained, mobility, flexibility and overall career aspirations of the individual. A Physician with a well-structured strategic career plan may benefit greatly from enrollment to an MBA course.

Physicians, like other potential MBA students, should establish the rationale for engaging into such an academic commitment. Many people appear to enroll into MBA courses without a clear career strategy for embarking on this route. Unfortunately, some MBA students are disappointed that their career is not accelerated. The reason for this is likely due to the fact that the MBA was not the remedial action required to resurrect a career that veered into an undesirable direction. However, once you have a clear rationale, then your choice of business school, duration and depth of study, cost and academic concentrations should become more obvious.

One of my own drivers for studying for the MBA was to remove the stigma of being a 'Physician' in industry. An initial perception of Physicians is that they are not expected to be strong in commercial or business management. Therefore, the MBA serves to marginalise that potential misperception. Conversely, Physicians, who are usually academically talented, can erroneously assume that their clinical competencies can be extrapolated into the Pharmaceutical and Corporate environment with little effort. This latter point can be a major mistake and can lead to serious career missteps, both of which can be mitigated by attaining the MBA. The MBA offers the Physician skill sets that are not provided in medical school curricula. These areas include organisational management, leadership, accounting, finance, strategy and marketing (Section 3).

PRIVATE HEALTHCARE

There are many examples of doctors with MBAs acting as Medical Directors and Commercial Directors throughout private healthcare insurers and providers, such as Bupa, Circle and Care UK. As the market for private healthcare in the UK opens up, there are likely to be increasing opportunities for medics as 'boundroids' (Box 16.3).

Andrew Vallance-Owen, Group Medical Director of Bupa, completed his MBA with the Open University whilst working for the British Medical Association (BMA). After completing his MBA, Andrew was invited to apply for the role of Medical Director for Bupa Hospitals. Andrew does not feel that the MBA was the most significant factor in helping him to secure this role. But Andrew did find his MBA helpful on a practical basis once in post at Bupa. He feels the most useful learning was about psychological theories of people management, discussed in Chapter 7: 'Medical training teaches you how to communicate with patients but less about how to communicate with your team'.

Andrew sees his greatest strength as being a medics' medic who is also able to understand the commercial side of healthcare. Being able to transition between and relate to both medical and corporate worlds, understanding and relating to the values of each, is one of the core advantages to being a medic with an MBA.

Mark Hunt is Managing Director of Healthcare, at Care UK, a leading independent provider of health and social care. The influence of doing an MBA on his career path is illustrated in Box 16.3.

BOX 16.3 Being a boundroid

Dr Mark Hunt, Managing Director of Healthcare, Care UK

It is a common understanding that the MBA only gets you the first job after your degree and after that it is down to your success in the next job that defines where you end up. However, it is 20 years since I completed an MBA and I am still drawing on the understanding.

An MBA gives you a structured approach to problem solving – it is good at developing the analytics and right brain stuff. It gives you the confidence for tackling the unknown. Medical training is technocratic and as a generalisation leads to a pattern of behaviour that means we have to know everything before we do anything and the MBA changes that to pattern recognition and to satisfying behaviour.

All this however is half the story – 'sweating the soft stuff' is the other ingredient for success. Part of the reason for the MBA being the route only to the next job is because it is a technical degree and the importance of knowledge diminishes as you progress in your career. Knowledge of self and leadership is the key to making an impact in bigger roles. The MBA does help in these areas and the knowledge for these areas can be learnt, i.e. leaders are not just born (see Chapter 7). The average age of MBA students is 27 and the developmental level for these students means the impact of the soft stuff is less. MBAs are structured around

(continued)

group working, and this provides an action-learning environment for testing some of your softer skills. However, there is no resting on your laurels; the MBA isn't the golden bullet, it is just the start of the journey.

As ever, it depends on what you ultimately want to do when you grow up after being an eternal student. The MBA by its very nature is a route to generalism and a variable opportunity to specialise according to the exact degree. I have always, unfashionably, enjoyed being a generalist, hence my choice of career as a GP. The MBA fed that interest, providing general management training and has led to my current role as Managing Director of a health and social care company employing 15 000 employees and a turnover of £410 million. Three of us are just undertaking a management buyout of the company.

The MBA gives, and gave me, the commercial insight, in a largely non commercial NHS. It marks a difference and a potential advantage compared to the other people that you work with. It has helped me to make the right decision, even though the rest of the people you work with don't see it. Personally it changed my outlook culturally; I use a different lens. You are, in The King's Fund terminology, 'a boundroid', and this helps in understanding which way up the world is, but beware – other people won't see it that way.

Career paths for technical people such as medics aren't clear. There are limited acceptable opportunities and incentives outside of training and the colleges. My career path has largely been by chance. In the main, I have been approached by colleagues and friends and asked to do the next job. The common thread in all of my jobs has been the difference in knowledge and outlook the MBA has given me and is the reason people have asked me to do the next job. Don't miss out but be clear why you choose to do an MBA as you won't be able to go back.

'THE CITY'

Although the glamour and prestige of working in 'the city' has been tarnished with the downfall of Lehman Brothers and Enron, amongst others, once bestowed with an MBA, you remain ideally placed to secure a highly paid role working in finance in the 'golden mile' of the city.

However, the breadth of chapters included in this book is indicative of the breadth of skills that individuals who do MBAs will have. Therefore, a financial job in 'the city' will not be suitable or preferable for all. Popular finance MBA destinations include investment banking, equity (capital or debt) markets, asset management, private wealth management (including stock broking) and private equity. Of these, private equity is the hardest for medics with MBAs to enter. Very few people are hired without prior experience of banking or corporate finance. Private equity firms tend to be reluctant to train people up. In addition, this sector has been hiring less since the credit crunch.

The entry level depends on the business school, as discussed in Section 2. MBA graduates from Harvard, Wharton, Stanford, Chicago, LBS or INSEAD would be able to enter financial roles as an associate. Those with an MBA from a lesser school are more likely to enter at a third-year analyst position. Classically, individuals will do two or three years as an analyst before being promoted to an associate. Analysts do not manage anyone because they are effectively at the bottom of the ladder. Generally, the associates manage the analysts. The vice presidents sit one level above the associates and probably do more of the active managing. The associates do more of the supervision and training of analysts.

SUMMARY

In as much as there is a wide range of individual motivations for doing an MBA, the outcomes are even more varied. This final chapter provides ideas for future career paths for medics with MBAs who aspire to diversify beyond direct clinical contact with patients, peppered by the stories of inspiring individuals. There are many more in addition to the above list. For example, medico-legal and medico-political career paths do not require an MBA. However, given their competitive nature an MBA may offer an additional CV asset, albeit an expensive one.

The skills of clinicians, particularly those with the ability to be lateral thinkers, are in much demand by other industries as well as healthcare. At present there is a shortage of clinicians with MBAs. However, doing an MBA is just the beginning. It is our hope that this book will inspire clinicians to use the frameworks and ideas it contains to bring improvement and benefit to patient care.

FURTHER READING

Gabriel K (2003). *Vault Career Guide to Sales and Trading*. New York: Vault Reports.

Harrison Careers Service (2010). *101 Choices in Finance*. www.harrisoncareers.com/index.asp

Schlossberg A, Gorelik A (2002). *Vault Career Guide to Investment Management*. New York: Vault Reports.

Index